THE HISTORY OF RADIOLOGY

IN SCOTLAND

1896–2000

THE HISTORY OF RADIOLOGY

IN SCOTLAND

1896–2000

John F Calder
Consultant Radiologist
Victoria Infirmary
Glasgow

DUNEDIN ACADEMIC PRESS
EDINBURGH

Published by
Dunedin Academic Press
Hudson House
8 Albany Street, Edinburgh EH1 3QB

ISBN 1 903765 05 6

British Library Cataloguing in Publication Data

A catalogue record for this book is available from
the British Library

Typeset by Trinity Typing
Printed in Great Britain by Polestar, Aberdeen

Contents

		Page
	Foreword	vi
	Introduction	vii
	List of Illustrations	ix
1	The Pioneers	1
2	Glasgow	9
3	Edinburgh	35

Illustrations

4	Aberdeen and Grampian	56
5	Dundee and Tayside	65
6	The Rest of Scotland	70
7	The Scottish Radiological Society	82
8	Current Resources	87
	Appendix I	
	Scottish Radiological Society Office Bearers	93
	AppendixII	
	Radiologists in Scotland, Present and Past	94
	Bibliography	107
	Index	113

Foreword

In 1895, Röntgen discovered x-rays. Within a few weeks Lord Kelvin had received a letter from Röntgen which he passed on to a relative and colleagues. By February 1896, an x-ray demonstration in Glasgow was arranged, shortly followed by the establishment of the world's first x-ray service to patients! The speed of acceptance of a revolutionary new physics principle was quite extraordinary as was the rapid development for investigating patients. No ethical committees nor long complicated review processes for scientific papers occurred in those days!

The rest is history; and this history has now been complied by John Calder, a well respected Scottish Radiologist who has produced this fascinating account of Radiology in Scotland. He has shown the considerable historical importance of Scotland's role in the development of 'Imaging' throughout the 20th Century.

The archive material has been obtained from numerous sources that have often produced new light on forgotten exploits. Scotland has had more than its fair share of world renowned figures in 'Radiology' and this text is a memento to their dedication, expertise and brilliance in their chosen fields. John Calder has managed, very effectively, to capture for posterity, the Scottish scene during the last 105 years since that momentous day in November 1895 when one of humanity's greatest discoveries was made.

J Weir
Chairman Standing Scottish Committee — Royal College of Radiologists
Past Dean and Vice President — Royal College of Radiologists

Introduction

The concept of writing the history of radiology in Scotland came from the 1995 Röntgen Centenary Congress in Birmingham. I had written the chapter on radiology in Scotland in "The Invisible Light" edited by Adrian Thomas and published to coincide with the centenary. In the process I had gathered more information than could be included in a short chapter and the possibility of writing a book began to emerge. The end of a millennium and the Scottish NHS trust mergers which were taking place simultaneously made the timing appropriate, especially as many of the hospitals in which most radiologists spent their working lives are likely to disappear in their present form. It was also an appropriate time to approach retired radiologists whose memories reach back to the beginning of the health service and before that source of information is lost.

Thanks to the prompting of Dr J K Davidson and the encouragement of my fellow council members of the Scottish Radiological Society, a decision was taken which was to culminate in the writing of this book. After several false starts when first a historian then a retired journalist were unable to do it for different reasons, I decided to undertake the task myself. This was more daunting than it first seemed, including as it did an information gathering exercise which has taken the best part of three years. How successful this has been will be for the reader to judge.

I could not have written the book without the help of radiologists and archivists from throughout Scotland. To a large extent, the information given about any particular hospital is a reflection of the enthusiasm and co-operation I have received from at least one present or retired radiologist.

While it would be invidious to name all those who have helped me in this project, I should like to single out a few for special mention. The radiologists are Jake Davidson, Lewis Gillanders, James Duncan, Tom Cowie, Lockhart Frain-Bell, Malcolm Merrick, John Bell, Sandy Robertson, Winton McNab, Monty Hadley, Allan Reid, Ken Brown, Roddy Cameron, Bill Gibson, Ruth MacKenzie, Alastair Kirkpatrick, Lind McDonald, David Nichols, Ian Riach, Bobby Corbett, Hilary Dobson, Jonathan Best and Jamie Weir. The radiotherapists are Gerry Robertson, Hugh McDougall, Mumtaz Elia and Tarun Sarkar. Bill Copland was responsible for most of the chapter on the Scottish Radiological Society with only the later additions contributed by me. Harry Gray provided the information on nuclear medicine in Glasgow Royal Infirmary and John Fleming contributed the history of ultrasound. I should also like to thank Alistair Tough and Mike Barfoot, archivists in Glasgow and Edinburgh respectively, and Laura Adam of the Department of Medicine in Dundee. No acknowledgement would be complete without giving thanks to my wife, Marion, for her support not only in this project but throughout my career.

This book is dedicated to the Scottish Radiological Society which I am proud to have served as President.

Illustrations

following page 55

1. The Author. John F Calder (President of the Scottish Radiological Society 1997–1999).

   Courtesy of the Department of Medical Illustrations, Victoria Infirmary, Glasgow

2. John Macintyre. Glasgow Royal Infirmary, 1895–1926.

3. X-ray room. Glasgow Royal Infirmary, 1896.

4. Macintyre's first x-ray of pulmonary tuberculosis.

5. John Macintyre. Commemorative plaque. Glasgow Royal Infirmary.

   2, 3, 4 and 5 reproduced by courtesy of Bill Paterson, Director of Medical Illustrations, Glasgow Royal Infirmary

6. James R Riddell. Glasgow Royal Infirmary, 1902–1920; Western Infirmary, 1920–1932.

7. The new x-ray department, Western Infirmary, Glasgow 1930.

8. X-ray room Western Infirmary 1930.

   7 & 8 reproduced from The Western Infirmary 1874–1974 by Loudon McQueen and Archibald B Kerr

9. Opening of the new x-ray department, Western Infirmary, 1930.
Sir John Roxburgh   Sir Brian Kelly   Col Mackintosh
Miss Smith
Mrs McCredie   Mrs R D McGregor   Lady Nairn

10. Prof Ian Donald scanning his daughter and grandchild.

7, 8, 9 and 10 reproduced by courtesy of Dr J K Davidson

11. Glasgow Campaign Against Tuberculosis.

Reproduced from Glasgow's X-Ray Campaign Against Tuberculosis. Glasgow Corporation, 1957

12. Sir George Beatson. Cancer Surgeon, Glasgow.

13. Dawson Turner's radiograph of a purse containing a florin and key, 1896.

Reproduced by kind permission of the President and Council of the Royal College of Surgeons of Edinburgh

Heads of Department at the Royal Infirmary of Edinburgh.

14. Dawson Turner 1898–1925

15. J Woodburn Morison 1926–1930

16. A E Barclay 1936

17. Duncan White 1930–1937

18. Robert McWhirter 1937–1945

19. W S Shearer 1946–1957

20. Eric Samuel 1958–1978

21. Tom Philp 1978–1986

14–21 reproduced by courtesy of the Department of Medical Illustration, Edinburgh Royal Infirmary.

22. John Paton McGibbon. Royal Infirmary of Edinburgh, 1942–1952.

23. George Pirie. Dundee Royal Infirmary, 1896–1925.

24. Martyrs' memorial, Hamburg showing the names of James R Riddell and George Pirie.

25. X-ray room, Lochmaben Sanatorium, 1927. The room had previously been the kitchen.

    Reproduced by courtesy of Dr L Frain-Bell

26. X-ray room, Queen Margaret Hospital, Dunfermline, 1949.

    Reproduced by courtesy of the Carnegie Museum, Dunfermiline

27. John Innes. Victoria Infirmary, Glasgow 1946–1972.

    Courtesy of the Department of Medical Illustrations, Victoria Infirmary, Glasgow

28. Robert Steiner (Royal College of Radiologists), Edward McGirr (Royal College of Physicians and Surgeons of Glasgow), Howard Middlemiss (Royal College of Radiologists) and Hunter Cummack (Scottish Radiological Society) at the establishment of the Standing Scottish Committee.

29. Some notable Scottish radiologists at a meeting in Glasgow, March 1985.
    Tony Brewin   Bill Duncan   Mike Buist   Jake Davidson
    Lewis Gillanders TonyDonaldson Bill Ross Gerry Flatman

30. X-Ray staff Southern General Hospital, Glasgow, June 1963.
    Wilson James, Jake Davidson and Kenneth Grossart are in the front row.

31. Western Infirmary, Glasgow x-ray staff at Ellis Barnett's retiral in January 1987.
    Back row: Hilary Dobson Alan Ramsay John Roberts John Straiton Colin Campbell Richard Edwards Sutherland McKechnie R Mahraj J Namasivayam
    Middle Row: Brian Mucci Fiona Howie Anne Hollman George Stenhouse Nigel McMillan Patricia Morley Michael Cowan Barbara Dall Susan Ingram Wilma Kincaid Grace Hare
    Front Row: Ramsay Vallance J McDermid Dorothy Rigg Ellis Barnett Jake Davidson R McKinnon Albert Aylmer Fred Adams

    28–31 reproduced by courtesy of Dr J K Davidson

32. Glasgow Royal Infirmary staff at J G Duncan's retiral in 1987.
    Back row: Fat Wui Poon Russell Pickard Allan Reid Patrick Walsh
    Middle row: Fiona Gardner Julian Guse Alastair Forrester Grant Baxter Michael Dean Ian McLeod Jean Lauder
    Front Row: Derek Lightbody Dorothy Anderson Nimmo McKellar James Duncan Brian Moule Ian Stewart

    Reproduced by courtesy of Dr A W Reid

32. Scottish Radiological Society Röntgen Centenary Dinner, Stirling Castle, 11th Nov. 1995.

    Reproduced by kind permission of Kodak Ltd

1

The Pioneers

The discovery of x-rays by Wilhelm Conrad Röntgen in November 1895 in Wurzburg has been chronicled elsewhere and is not the subject of this book. It is the link between Röntgen and the early introduction of radiology to Scotland which is relevant.

In the first week of 1896 Röntgen sent offprints of his paper to two distinguished British physicists: Professor Arthur Shuster in Manchester and Lord Kelvin in Glasgow. Kelvin was considered at that time to be the doyen of European physicists.

A copy of Kelvin's reply to Röntgen has been preserved and is as follows:

"Dear Prof Röntgen

When I wrote to you thanking you for your kindness in sending me your paper and the photographs which accompanied it I had only seen the photographs and had not had time to read the paper.

I need not tell you that when I read the paper I was very much astonished and delighted. I can say no more just now than to congratulate you warmly on the great discovery you have made and to renew my thanks to you for your kindness in so early sending me your paper and the photographs.

Believe me,

Yours very truly,

Kelvin"

Kelvin was ill at the time he received the paper and so he passed it to his brother-in-law Dr J T Bottomley who was associated with Lord Blythswood and Dr John Macintyre in electrical experiments. These three gave the first demonstration of x-rays in Glasgow to the Philosophical Society on 5th February 1896.

John Macintyre

John Macintyre was born to Donald and Margaret Macintyre at 343 High Street, Glasgow, near the Royal Infirmary on 2nd October 1857. His mother was a first cousin of explorer and missionary David Livingstone.

Macintyre was educated at the local school in Townhead and left at the age of 11 because he suffered from severe headaches. Between leaving school and entering university he took several jobs and studied electrical engineering. At the age of 21 he entered Glasgow University as a medical student and graduated MB CM with commendation in 1882 at the age of 25.

After graduation, he studied in London, Paris and Vienna and also made a voyage to India as a ship's surgeon.

His first interest was in ear, nose and throat surgery and in this capacity he was appointed assistant surgeon at Glasgow Royal Infirmary in 1886 and full surgeon in 1893.

He had been appointed medical electrician to Glasgow Royal Infirmary in 1885 and was responsible for equipping the hospital with electrical current for medical and surgical purposes. The wards and operating theatres were wired throughout. At this time the streets of Glasgow were still gas-lit.

Macintyre became a council member of the British Laryngological, Rhinological and Otological Association in 1893 and vice president in 1900. For many years he was proprietor and editor of the Journal of Laryngology. He set up a consultant practice in his rooms at 179 Bath Street. As an eminent ENT surgeon he was consulted by and befriended many of the leading performers of the day including Paderewski, Sir Henry Irvine, Dame Nellie Melba, Luiza Tetrazzini, the novelist Joseph Conrad, and Thomas Eddison. Macintyre made recordings of the voices of many of his famous guests on phonograph wax cylinders. Unfortunately none of these recordings survives, as they melted in the heat of his attic.

However, it is as a medical electrician that Macintyre is best known. In collaboration with Dr J T Bottomley and Lord Blythswood and with the assistance of Lord Kelvin in providing apparatus which he would not have obtained otherwise, Macintyre produced a radiograph by the Röntgen method.

It is difficult to ascertain who was responsible for producing the first radiograph in Britain. Campbell Swinton, a Scottish electrical consultant, who had moved to London, is generally credited with being the first. He produced a radiograph of his own hand on 13th January 1896. A photograph of his hand was published in Nature on 23rd January 1896.

By this time, Macintyre had already given a lecture in Glasgow University to doctors and students on "The New Light". The first documented public presentation of Macintyre's work was presented jointly by Bottomley, Blythswood and Macintyre to the Philosophical Society of Glasgow on "The Röntgen Rays" or "The New Photography" on 5th February 1896. It is remarkable that Macintyre enunciated what are still today the principles of good radiography only five weeks after Lord Kelvin had received Röntgen's paper. In March 1996 only a month after his address to the Philosophical Society, Macintyre obtained permission of the managers of the Royal Infirmary to form a new branch of the electrical department. Despite the controversy which exists about who took the first x-ray in Britain, few would dispute that Macintyre's was the first x-ray department in the world to provide a service to patients. The many "firsts" which can be attributed to Macintyre include the first radiological demonstration of a bullet, the first of a renal calculus, the first radiographs of thorax and abdomen, the first radiograph of a tuberculous hip, the first of a coin in the oesophagus and the first demonstration of breast cancer by x-rays. Perhaps the most spectacular of his innovations was the production of a ciné-radiograph of a moving frog's leg. Copies of this film exist in the Royal College of Physicians and Surgeons of Glasgow and the Scottish Film Archive.

Silvanus Thompson, first President of the Röntgen Society, in his presidential address in 1897, said, "To particularise might be invidious but none will object to my mention of the name of Dr Macintyre of Glasgow ... who was one of the earliest and most successful practitioners of the new art".

Like other early medical electricians, Macintyre took an interest in the treatment of patients by x-rays. He also established a radium department in the Royal Infirmary.

Early in his career, Macintyre observed that skin reactions were common, thus recognising the dangers of x-rays. Because of his awareness of these dangers he was not, unlike many other pioneers, a martyr to radiology. John Scott, his distinguished chief radiographer, wrote, "Macintyre was very strict on the question of protection, both of patients and of staff". He also described Macintyre as a man with restless energy but who was also frank, sagacious, unaffected, and genial with a ready wit and charming personality.

John Macintyre received many honours. He was President of the Röntgen Society, a Deputy Lieutenant of Glasgow, and an LLD of Glasgow University. He was created a Knight of Grace of the Order of St John and was elected a Fellow of the Royal Society of Edinburgh. John Macintyre died after a short illness at the age of 73 on 29th October 1928 in his native city of Glasgow.

Dawson Turner

Dawson Turner was born in Liverpool in 1857. He graduated from Dalhousie University in Canada, then came to Edinburgh in 1884. He graduated MB CM with honours in 1888 and MD in 1890. Following house jobs in Edinburgh, he studied in Oxford, Paris and Vienna before returning to Edinburgh to lecture in physics at Surgeons' Hall. Before 1895 he was already the author of several works on medical electricity in diagnosis and treatment. He was therefore in a good position to recognise the importance of the announcement of Röntgen's discovery of x-rays. He set up a primitive apparatus in his house at 37 George Street where his neighbour was Peter Tait, Professor of Natural Philosophy at the University of Edinburgh and a close collaborator with Sir William Thompson, afterwards Lord Kelvin.

Dawson Turner demonstrated photographs taken by the Röntgen process to a meeting of the Edinburgh Medico-Chirurgical Society on 5th February 1896 with Dr Argyle Robertson in the chair.

In November 1896 Robert Milne Murray was appointed medical electrician with Turner as his assistant. Murray became a gynaecologist in 1901 which left Turner in charge until his partial retirement in 1911. After 1911 he was "extra" electrician till 1925.

Turner did not escape the physical disabilities suffered by early radiation workers and sustained severe radiation burns which eventually caused the loss of three fingers and an eye. He died on Christmas Day 1928.

James Mackenzie Davidson

James Mackenzie Davidson was born in Buenos Aires of Scots parents and received his early education at the Scottish school there. He studied medicine in Edinburgh, London and Aberdeen and graduated MB CM from Aberdeen in 1882. He made his career in ophthalmology and succeeded Professor Dyce Davidson as ophthalmic surgeon to Aberdeen Royal Infirmary in 1886.

Through his interest in physics and his leisure time experiments in electricity and light, he was quick to realise the potential for the use of the newly discovered x-rays in ophthalmology. When Röntgen published his paper in 1896 Mackenzie Davidson went to Wurzburg to interview him and find out all he could about the new discovery. He is another to have a claim on being among the first in Scotland to produce photographs using x-rays.

As an ophthalmologist he realised the value of x-rays in demonstrating foreign bodies in the eye. He developed the Mackenzie Davidson localiser, a stereoscopic device for locating these foreign bodies. This apparatus will always be associated with him.

In 1897, like many other Scots before and since, he decided to pursue his career in London. In the same year he published a radiograph of a bladder stone demonstrating that his interest in radiology had encompassed areas other than ophthalmology.

His London career is not part of the history of radiology in Scotland but it should be recorded that he became Britain's leading radiologist in the first decade of the twentieth century and was knighted for his achievements in 1912. He died of heart failure on 2nd April 1919.

George Pirie

Soon after their discovery, interest in x-rays was taken both at University College, Dundee and at Dundee Royal Infirmary. By

1886 the first report on x-rays from the city had been published. The early experimental work was carried out by Professor Waymouth Reid, professor of physiology, and Professor Johannes Kuenen, professor of physics who shared an interest in x-rays which must have started soon after the first reports from Germany were available. In March 1896 they wrote to the Council of University College seeking extra funds for their research work. In 1897 Waymouth Reid subjected himself to four exposures of up to 20–90 minutes duration within a period of four days. This resulted in severe dermatitis and loss of hair for a prolonged period with effects on his chest and back. Without any appreciation of the risks, further experiments were undertaken involving not only themselves but others. Reid records in his observations: "Passage of the rays for an hour through the head of a laboratory boy of medium intelligence did not in my hands cause deterioration or improvement thereof". No ethical committee today would approve the use of a laboratory boy "of whatever intelligence" as a subject for such experiments. However, it is possible but by no means certain that had the serious side effects been appreciated, progress in developing the clinical application of x-rays might have been abandoned or at best delayed.

Dr George Pirie was appointed honorary medical electrician to Dundee in 1896, established the first electrical department at the Royal Infirmary that year, and published his first clinical picture in 1897. By the turn of the century radiology was developing quickly and expanding as a clinical speciality. Pirie faced a problem in the early 1900s no different from his colleagues today. His notes submitted to meetings of directors of the Royal Infirmary (in 1911 and 1913) set out his requirements for x-ray diagnosis:

1 Sufficient fresh plates delivered promptly
2 Sufficient x-ray lamps each month
3 A trained electrical mechanic
4 Efficient apparatus free from danger
5 Plates to be properly developed
6 A nurse to help the patients
7 A senior resident to help me

In 1913 Pirie wrote to his colleagues in established departments in the larger cities seeking factual advice and comment. Replies from three have been preserved — from James Riddell in Glasgow, Thurston Holland in Liverpool, and Archibald McKendrick in Edinburgh. He sought the following information:

1 The title of their appointment(s)
2 Their responsibilities
3 Their fees
4 The hours of work
5 The workload
6 Level of supporting staff
7 Wages paid

Their replies gave a good example of a typical workload of the day (see pages 10 and 35).

Pirie himself had carried out 1,260 examinations in 1909.

In 1905 there is the first record of Pirie developing skin trouble which started as dryness and cracking and progressed to skin tumours. His hands were exposed constantly to x-rays. The use of the hand fluoroscope to check tube output and image quality was a source of considerable radiation. A bottle of mustard oil which he used to soothe his hands, has been preserved. Eventually his health failed. He had lost fingers and of necessity had to resign his post in 1925. In the end he lost both hands.

His contribution to medical care in Dundee and the suffering he endured in consequence were recognised. When forced to give up work he was awarded a Civil List Pension and a Carnegie Hero Trust Medal and Pension. Dundee City Council opened a public subscription and in 1926 he was presented with an award of £1,120 in grateful recognition of his services.

Pirie died in October 1929 aged 66 years and is buried in the Western Cemetery in Dundee.

He is commemorated on the Hamburg Memorial as one of the radiologists from all over the world who became martyrs to the development of radiology. The memorial which stands in the grounds of St George's Radiotherapy Hospital, Hamburg, was unveiled in 1836. On the memorial there are the names of 169 radiologists from 14 countries. There are seven from Scotland: William Hope Fowler, Edinburgh; J W L Spence, Edinburgh; Dawson Turner, Edinburgh; John Hall Edward, Edinburgh;

James Riddell, Glasgow; George Pirie, Dundee; William Ironside Bruce, Aberdeen and London.

2

Glasgow

The Royal Infirmary

As described in the opening chapter, John Macintyre was responsible for establishing at the Royal Infirmary an x-ray department which has good claims to have been the first in the world. A summary in 1902 of his own technical description of the department is as follows: "The installation may be divided into three distinct components. Firstly, the rooms themselves are lighted by the 250 volt circuit from the Corporation; secondly, a transformer has been built by Messrs Mavor & Coulson to give 55 volts and 50 amperes from the Corporation supply; thirdly, there is the old gas engine, with dynamo and secondary cells, giving 56 volts and 30 amperes. The last two are intended for all medical and surgical purposes, whether for diagnostic or therapeutic use, and by means of turn-over switches can be used, so that, in the event of a breakdown with the Corporation supply through the transformer, the gas engine and cells can be utilised and vice versa. For x-rays, three large coils capable of giving 14 to 12 inches spark respectively, have been added to the installation. All the well-known forms of interrupters have been fitted up, including the mercury, Mackenzie Davidson and Wehnelt. A specially designed switchboard has been attached to the wall, with rheostats for motors, volt and ampere meters. There is also a special set of switches, so that any one of the interrupters with suitable condensers can be instantly employed as required for different purposes. Stands and vacuum tubes (Queen's, Dean's and Cox's record designs) have been provided, as well as fluorescent screens, and all the most recent accessories for therapeutic as well as photographic purposes. Two couches have been provided for taking photographs from above or from below. There is also a localiser for detecting the situation of foreign bodies. All the apparatus necessary for the taking and demonstration of stereoscopic photographs has been added to the department".

James Robertson Riddell joined Macintyre, initially as his assistant, in 1899. He was born in Glasgow in 1873, the son of the Rev John Riddell of the Wynd Church. He received his medical education at the Royal Infirmary and obtained the Scottish triple qualification in 1897. In addition to his work at the Royal, he built up a large radiological practice and was considered the leading x-ray specialist in Glasgow. He was asked to superintend the establishment of radiological departments in many west of Scotland hospitals and to act as consultant. These hospitals included the Eye Infirmary, the Royal Hospital for Sick Children and the Royal Alexandra Infirmary, Paisley. In a letter to James Pirie of Dundee, written from his home and consulting room at 1 Royal Crescent, Glasgow in 1913, Riddell replies:

"Dear Dr Pirie,
I work at the Royal Infirmary (roughly) two hours every day except Sunday 9am to 11am. I have two medical assistants at £25 each being there two hours daily — the one 9–11 and the other 11–1 but we do no treatment without a medical present in the department hence the two assists. We have a young man who does the routine work of taking skiagrams in the wards and smaller things such as hands and legs, and he develops all the skias. We have a Sister and five Nurses (I think by arrangement we could do with less). Last year x-ray exams numbered about 6,600 a number being repeats and duplicates (say to the extent of 1,200). The Directors of the Royal Cancer Hospital have asked me to take the job there and I have agreed. I expect to do less than half there (perhaps 1/4) and get an hon. of £25. I expect to have a nurse to assist me. Any information I can give I shall do with great pleasure.
Yours sincerely,
James R Riddell"

This must be the first (and last) example of any radiologist admitting that he could manage with fewer staff!

At the outbreak of the Great War, Riddell saw service in the east and at Salonika with the rank of Major and became x-ray expert to the Scottish Command. On taking up his post at the Western Infirmary in 1920, he relinquished his other hospital appointments.

Details about the Royal x-ray department between the wars are not well recorded and merit only a brief paragraph in "The History of the Royal Infirmary 1792–1994". This book does record that the x-ray department continued to provide a valuable asset but also a heavy drain on the Infirmary's funds. Over 26,000 examinations were carried out each year, consuming up to £5,000 per annum for film alone. The equipment was very expensive, due to high protective tariffs on foreign imports during the 1930s, and it was pointed out to delegates of the working-class contributors in 1935 that, whereas John Macintyre was able to purchase an x-ray tube for thirty shillings during the 1890s, the price of modern tubes had risen to £200 each.

It is known that the medical electricians during this period were Katherine Chapman (1920–24), Bruce MacLean (1925–26), Donald Livingston Macintyre (1923–39), Alan Balfour Black (1923–40) and Robert Crawford (1927–40). In addition to his Royal Infirmary appointments Balfour Black was in charge of the two Glasgow Corporation hospitals, Stobhill and the Southern General and it is mainly with Stobhill that he is associated. Robert Crawford also held an appointment at the Southern General until he retired in 1960. Donald Macintyre was the son of John Macintyre and is the first Scottish example of a son following his father into radiology. There are other examples of daughters and sons who have followed their fathers. They are Elspeth Lindsay (Crosshouse) and Barbara Macpherson (Law), daughters of Peter Macpherson (Institute of Neurological Sciences); Fiona Gilbert (Aberdeen), daughter of J K Davidson (Western, Glasgow); Fiona Howie (Hairmyres), daughter of Harry Gardner (Victoria, Glasgow) and Donald Hadley (Institute of Neurological Sciences), son of Monty Hadley (Inverness).

Robert Kemp Harper was director of radiology at the Royal from 1939 to 1946, when he left to take charge of the department in St. Bartholomew's Hospital. He became Vice President of the Faculty of Radiologists from 1950–51. Other radiologists who worked at the Royal at this time were Mrs M C Leishman, Robert Klein and Anthony Vickers. Eugene Timoshenko, a Russian emigré who adopted the name Calder, was a consultant from

1942 to 1969. He took a particular interest in cardiac radiology and was by all accounts a man with a formidable reputation. When the author started training in the Royal in 1971 he was often asked if they were related. They are not.

James Zuill Walker became director of diagnostic radiology in 1947. He was educated at Hillhead High School, Glasgow and graduated MB ChB from the University of Glasgow in 1930. He obtained the DMRE, Cambridge in 1933 and the FFR in 1937. After appointments at the Victoria Infirmary, Glasgow, Edinburgh Royal Infirmary and as medical director of Lincolnshire Cancer Organisation, he was appointed to the Royal. At the same time, he was radiologist in charge of x-ray services in West Lanarkshire, a post which he did not relinquish till 1965. He was in charge of the department at the beginning of the National Health Service. Because of his expertise, he became closely associated with the development of diagnostic radiology in other hospitals within the Western Region. Dr Walker's strongly held views on radiology were not always acceptable to his colleagues. Nevertheless his integrity was such that he was held universally in the highest esteem. His colleagues admired his courage and fortitude in working to shortly before his death, giving no indication to other than his immediate family that he was dying of prostatic carcinoma.

Other consultant radiologists appointed during Jim Walker's time in charge were Sidney Haase in 1950, David Raeside in 1950, Nimmo McKellar in 1963 and Brian Moule in 1966. Sidney Haase is better known as head of department in Stobhill Hospital after he left the Royal.

David Raeside had responsibilities in Belvidere Hospital as well as at the Royal. Nimmo McKellar brought considerable skills as a vascular radiologist from the Institute of Neurological Sciences, then situated at Killearn Hospital. He was well respected by consultants throughout the hospital and by several generations of registrars who benefited from his wisdom and experience. It was through his association with the department of respiratory medicine that pulmonary angiography was brought to the Royal, a mixed blessing for registrars on call! Brian Moule also carried out vascular procedures but is better known for bringing biliary radiology to the department. He developed percutaneous cholangiography and ERCP in conjunction with Prof Leslie Blumgart of the department of surgery. He also had responsibility for radiology in the facio-maxillary unit at Canniesburn Hospital.

James G Duncan was appointed consultant in administrative charge in 1969. He began his radiology training in Edinburgh in 1948 and obtained the DMRD within 18 months and the FFR in 1955. He became a consultant in Edinburgh in 1956 and, shortly before his appointment to the Royal, spent six months as visiting professor in the university department of radiology at the Strong Memorial Hospital, Rochester, New York. Between his appointment and his retiral in 1987, several important developments took place in the Royal. In addition to those in vascular and biliary radiology, the first NE 4101 scanner with its non-persistence oscilloscope was installed around 1971. The radiologist, usually a registrar, performed a compound B-scan while Sister Wallace took the image on a Polaroid camera before it faded. Many of the early scans were for pregnancy dating. Some of the registrars had obstetric experience and when the scan disagreed with their clinical estimate of gestation it was usually the latter they believed. In 1981 the Royal was the first Glasgow hospital apart from the Institute of Neurological Sciences to install a CT scanner. Along with David Meek, a senior registrar who subsequently went to Liverpool, Dr Duncan published work on computed tomography of liver metastases.

Derek Lightbody was appointed in 1969 and took over the cardiac interest from Dr Timoshenko. Patrick Fitzgerald Finch and S Yogarajah had relatively short spells as consultant radiologists before they left to become colleagues in Milton Keynes. Of the present radiologists, Dorothy Anderson and Ian Stewart were both appointed in 1981. Ian developed Brian Moule's interest in biliary radiology further into the interventional field.

In 1982 the long awaited move from the basement of the old medical block to phase one of the new hospital took place.

G Roberton ("Roy") Sutherland took over as consultant in administrative charge in 1987. He had trained in radiology in Edinburgh before being appointed consultant at the Southern General, Glasgow. He left the Southern to become consultant in administrative charge at Stobhill. When the two hospitals had a relatively short lived administrative merger, he took over at the Royal as well. The rapid pace of change continued and during his term of office both the vascular room and the CT scanner were replaced with the latest equipment.

Since Roy's retiral in 1991 changes in the ways that departments are run, the setting up of NHS trusts in 1994 and their subsequent mergers (still ongoing) into super trusts have caused more frequent changes in the directorship of x-ray departments. Who would have thought that those traditional rivals, the Royal and the Western (along with Stobhill) would merge into one administrative unit. It is unlikely that we have seen the end of these changes. Brian Moule became consultant in administrative charge in 1991 and clinical director in 1993. Subsequent clinical directors have been Alastair Forrester from 1995 to 1996 and Allan Reid from 1996 to 2000.

Of the radiologists appointed since 1987 Fat Wui Poon is the first to have formal sessions in nuclear medicine. Eddie Leen has particular research interests in hepatic liver disease and has published widely on the use of Doppler ultrasound in this respect. Allan Reid and Douglas McCarter both have a strong vascular interest and this has extended to MRI since the Royal's first scanner was installed in 1998. It is interesting that the Royal and Western have different approaches to interventional radiology. The Royal radiologists are system orientated, whereas those at the Western, while primarily vascular radiologists, cross system boundaries in their interventional techniques. For these and other reasons, attempts at providing a Glasgow wide on call rota for interventional radiology have failed so far. Janet Litherland has the main interest in breast radiology. Giles Roditi came from Aberdeen, one of the main centres to pioneer MRI. His knowledge of this has been invaluable in setting up the new scanning service.

The Royal Infirmary is one of only two centres in Scotland recognised for training in nuclear medicine. Its development has been in the hands of physicians rather than radiologists.

Edward McGirr, retired Muirhead Professor and Dean of the Faculty of Medicine is the doyen of Scottish nuclear medicine. After a short period of training at the Hammersmith Hospital London, he developed the first radioisotope service in Scotland at the Royal in the early 1950s. At that time the interests of the service were in the diagnosis and treatment of thyroid and blood disorders. He was succeeded in 1960 by Provan Murray who left for Sydney, Australia in 1963 to be replaced by John A Thomson. The service expanded with the addition of in vitro tests for total T4 estimations by competitive binding and the T3 resin sponge test. Thomson was one of the first in the UK to assess an early prototype of the EKCO gamma camera. The first isotope scanner at the Royal was commissioned in 1965 and imaged thyroid, brain and liver with isotopes of iodine, mercury and gold. When William Greig took over in 1967, "radioisotopes" became "nuclear medicine" and pertechnetate imaging became the norm.

Physics input at the Royal became established by the appointment of Lesley Hooper in 1966 and in 1972 Rodney Bessent arrived to lead the scientific staff in what had become a truly multidisciplinary department. Several young physicians began their training under Greig. Harry Gray and Ross McDougal were first, followed by Denis Citrin and James McKillop, now Muirhead Professor of Medicine. Later came Ignac Fogelman and Linda Smith. Drs McDougal, Gray and McKillop each trained in nuclear medicine in the USA in the early to late 1970s and greatly improved the academic credentials of the department. When Ross McDougal left permanently to work in Stanford, California and Bill Greig developed his final illness in the late 1970s, Harry Gray became consultant physician in charge of nuclear medicine. By 1980 nuclear cardiology had separated from nuclear medicine and has been run from within the department of cardiology since then. Nuclear medicine moved into custom-built premises in 1982 with the opening of the Queen Elizabeth Building. Since then the major research interests have been in venous thromboembolism, parathyroid disease and inflammatory bowel disease. Fat Wui Poon developed a link with radiology in 1990 and has sessions in both departments. Brian Neilly joined in 1994.

The Western Infirmary

The first medical electrician at the Western Infirmary was Donald J Mackintosh who, between the years of 1896 and 1920, combined the roles of medical superintendent and medical electrician. He was educated at Madras College, St. Andrews and at the University of Glasgow, where he graduated in 1884. His main interest was of necessity in areas which might be of clinical value, particularly skeletal radiology. He wrote a Skiagraphic Atlas of Fractures and Dislocations in 1899, one of the first radiological textbooks. A man with a dictatorial manner, he was said not to suffer fools gladly but hid a warm and kindly disposition and a keen sense of humour behind his forceful character. After the South African war he became MVO and for his work in the Great War he was made CB. He was also a Knight of Grace of the Order of St. John of Jerusalem. He was awarded an LLB by Glasgow University and was a Deputy Lieutenant of the County of the City of Glasgow.

In 1908 W F Somerville, Archibald Hay and J Goodwin Tomkinson were appointed medical electricians. Latterly, Tomkinson became much better known as a dermatologist but continued his interest in x-ray therapy as applied to diseases of the skin.

When Somerville and Hay retired in 1920, James R Riddell was appointed medical electrician and was also the first holder of the university lectureship in electrical diagnosis and therapeutics at the Western Infirmary. It is interesting to comment that while there is now a chair of radiotherapy and oncology in Glasgow, diagnostic radiology has never progressed to having a university department. Riddell provides a link between the Royal and Western Infirmaries in that he started his career in the Royal with John Macintyre and worked there for many years before being appointed to the Western. He was there at the time of many important advances: the replacement of x-ray plates by film, the development of the Coolidge tube and the introduction of contrast media and bismuth meals. He was particularly interested in the therapeutic aspects of radiology and contributed articles to medical journals on the use of x-rays in malignant disease, uterine fibroids and on the therapeutic aspects of radium. In 1923 it is recorded that x-ray therapy applications numbered 1,829, fluoroscopic examinations 3,899 and skiagrams 10,737. An assistant electrician, Laurence T Stewart was appointed to help with the increasing workload. Stewart died an untimely death only seven years later.

Like many other early radiologists, Riddell suffered from the effects of x-rays and had many operations to remove malignant growths. He resigned because of ill health and died on 29th June 1935.

In 1933 J Struthers Fulton succeeded James Riddell. Fulton began his medical studies in Edinburgh after serving in the Great

War. After some years in general practice, he returned to Edinburgh in 1930 and obtained a diploma in radiology with honours. This was followed by his MD and FRCP (Ed). He was assistant radiologist at Edinburgh Royal Infirmary until 1932 and was then invited to take charge of the deep x-ray department at the Holt Radium Institute, Manchester as a colleague of Ralston Paterson. Fulton spent six years at the Western. During this time much streamlining and automation was achieved in the 1930 single story building, still recognisable today despite the addition of many "temporary" outbuildings. The most up to date radiotherapy apparatus was installed and Fulton moved radiology strongly in the direction of radiotherapy. He recognised few therapeutic boundaries, treating tuberculous glands, carbuncles and aortic stenosis. He left the Western on his appointment as director of radiotherapy in Liverpool. He subsequently served with distinction in the Second World War, reaching the rank of Brigadier. He received a CBE for his services.

Fulton was succeeded in 1939 by Stanley Scott Park. Scott Park was born in Rhodesia and educated at Glasgow Academy and the University of Glasgow. He was influenced to take up radiology by James Riddell. They became life long friends and partners in private practice. Scott Park had the difficulty of maintaining an adequate service through the Second World War with a depleted and often temporary staff. During the blackout in November 1942 a fire caused by an electrical fault destroyed the radiotherapy transformer. Despite the difficulties caused by the incident it proved a blessing in disguise since apparatus approaching obsolescence had to be replaced by up to date equipment which would otherwise have been unobtainable in wartime. In 1946 radiotherapy and diagnostic radiology separated. This allowed Scott Park, better known as a clinical radiologist, to expand the diagnostic department. However, it was not until 1963 that he was able to take over the rooms which had been used by the radiotherapists.

Following the inauguration of the National Health Service in 1948 Scott Park became an adviser to the former Western Regional Hospital Board. He also became Vice President of the Faculty of Radiologists and President of the Scottish Radiological Society. Developments which took place while Scott Park was in charge included angiography in 1954 and ultrasound in 1963. In 1967, the year he retired, 62,185 patients had undergone radiological examinations.

Other notable radiologists at the Western in the latter part of Scott Park's time in charge and after his retirement were David Stenhouse, Tom Cowie and Ellis Barnett. While a medical registrar, the author was introduced to cardiac radiology by Tom Cowie and when his consultants asked him to obtain a radiological opinion, it was from Dr Stenhouse or Dr Barnett. Ellis Barnett carried out research into bone density in conjunction with the Bone and Calcium Metabolism Unit but is best known for his interest in ultrasound. This will be considered separately. He is also an excellent raconteur and in great demand as an after dinner speaker. David Stenhouse and Tom Cowie went to Gartnavel General Hospital when it opened in 1973, originally as a temporary measure while the Western was rebuilt. This did not happen and the redevelopment has never progressed beyond phase 1. The two departments now operate under a single clinical director.

In 1967 John Knight Davidson (better known to his contemporaries as "Jake") came from the Southern General to take charge at the Western. An Edinburgh graduate, he qualified on 5th July 1948, the day the National Health Service began. He trained in radiology in Edinburgh and St. Bartholomew's, London. Through his research and publications on aseptic necrosis of bone and decompression bone disease (the subject of his MD thesis) he became one of the best known Scottish radiologists both nationally and internationally. He was also known for his interest in adrenal venography in association with the MRC Blood Pressure Unit. Shortly before his retiral in 1990 Dr Davidson was awarded an OBE for his services to medicine. It is an interesting comment on the changes that have taken place since 1990 that some of the current generation of Glasgow registrars have been known to ask: "Who was Jake Davidson?".

The rapid developments of modern radiology allowed many advances, particularly in ultrasound and CT, to take place during "Jake's" years in charge and immediately afterwards. The rate of advance has only been slowed by the lack of finance available to develop the new technology.

Of the radiologists still in post, Frederick Adams joined the department in 1971 and was head of department for a short time after Dr Davidson's retiral. He developed a particular interest in nuclear medicine and was originally associated with Stewart Scott of the radiotherapy department in this venture. His other interests originally included vascular and interventional radiology which have now been taken further by Richard Edwards and Jonathan Moss. Richard developed an interest in interventional radiology while still a senior registrar and pursued many new techniques. His first consultant post was in Liverpool. Jon Moss was appointed vascular and interventional radiologist in 1992 and Richard later rejoined the department as consultant. Together they make a progressive and formidable interventional team. Ramsay Vallance who joined the department in 1977 was another with a vascular interest but he is now better known as gastro-intestinal radiologist and is the author of an "Atlas of Diagnostic Radiology in Gastroenterology", published by Blackwell in 1999. Laura Wilkinson holds a shared post with breast screening and has an interest in breast MRI.

Nigel McMillan was appointed in 1983 and followed Fred Adams as clinical director. He was involved in the development of CT and in MRI when the Western became the first general hospital in Glasgow to install a scanner in 1993. Nigel Raby joined him in this venture and is best known as a musculo-skeletal radiologist. He is co-author of "Accident and Emergency Radiology: a Survival Guide" published by W B Saunders in 1993. Michael Cowan, whose main interest is in cardiorespiratory radiology, followed Nigel McMillan as clinical director. George Stenhouse joined the department in 1981 from an academic background in physiology. As well as being an extremely well respected and hard working radiologist he is famous as an after dinner speaker and for giving extremely humorous votes of thanks to visiting speakers. Such is his reputation that it was difficult to find a successor as secretary to the Glasgow division of radiologists. Wilma Kincaid and Grant Baxter (mentioned later in the section on ultrasound) have interests in both ultrasound and CT.

Drs Vallance, Moss, Edwards, Wilkinson and Sinclair are now mainly based at Gartnavel General Hospital. Drs Cowan, Adams, Stenhouse, McMillan, Raby, Baxter and Kincaid are mainly at the Western.

Ultrasound. No history of imaging at the Western would be complete without a mention of ultrasound. The name which will always be associated with its early development is that of Ian Donald. He was born in Cornwall in 1910, the son and grandson of Scottish doctors. He was educated at Fettes College, Edinburgh and the universities of Cape Town and London, from which he graduated MB BS. Following medical service in the RAF and, later, academic posts in obstetrics at St. Thomas's and the Hammersmith Hospitals in London, he was appointed to the Regius Chair in Midwifery in Glasgow University in 1954.

Diagnostic ultrasound developed in Glasgow when Prof Donald was invited to the research department of boiler makers Babcock and Wilcox by one of their directors, the husband of a grateful patient. There he saw an A-scope industrial detector, the Kelvin Hughes Mark 4 and saw the possibilities of clinical application. In 1995 he obtained a second hand Kelvin Hughes Mark 2b "supersonic flaw detector" for the Western Infirmary. His association with Kelvin Hughes provides an interesting link with the earliest days of radiology in Scotland as it was Lord Kelvin, one of the founders of the company, who was first informed of Röntgen's work and stimulated John Macintyre's interest in medical electricity. In 1956 a young engineer from Kelvin Hughes, Tom Brown, introduced himself to Ian Donald and together with John McVicar, then a registrar, formed the team which was to develop first gynaecological then obstetric ultrasound. The first work on a 2D scanner took place in 1957 but the original results were still quite crude. In 1958 The Lancet published the report by Donald, McVicar and Brown, entitled "Investigation of abdominal masses by pulsed ultrasound". This article ranks as the most significant in the development of ultrasound in obstetrics and gynaecology. Following Kelvin Hughes' early involvement, many of the first commercial A and B scanners were Diasonographs, later taken over by Nuclear Enterprises of Edinburgh and finally by EMI. Further advances in real time scanning mainly took place in Japan, USA and continental Europe. Scotland, as in so many other developments which it pioneered, has become an importer rather than an exporter of ultrasonic equipment. Gynaecological ultrasound continued to develop at the Western and obstetric ultrasound at Glasgow Royal Maternity Hospital from 1959. It was not until

1964 that Ian Donald moved to the newly built Queen Mother's Hospital, adjacent to the Royal Hospital for Sick Children. Although the early work on ultrasound was done by obstetricians and gynaecologists, radiologists soon became involved and took ultrasound forward into the diverse clinical applications with which we are familiar today.

The first radiologist to take up ultrasound at the Western and the Royal Maternity was Ellis Barnett. He was joined later by Patricia Morley. They became among the best known names in British ultrasound and published an early textbook on the subject. Dr Barnett kindly donated his royalties from the first edition of their book to the Royal College of Radiologists to fund the Ellis Barnett prize in ultrasound. Their work has now been taken forward by others, notably Grant Baxter who is co-author (with Paul Allan of Edinburgh and Patricia Morley) of the second edition of Clinical Diagnostic Ultrasound, published by Blackwell in 1999.

Stobhill Hospital

From 1914 to 1925 x-ray films were made by the sister of Ward 13A under the supervision of Mr Cameron, a physics master at Allan Glen's school. In 1925 Dr A Balfour Black was the first radiologist to be appointed to Stobhill. He served in this capacity for the unusually long period of 36 years until he retired in 1960. In 1925 the original x-ray department shared with the physiotherapists a side room of Ward 13A. This small room was, not unnaturally, overcrowded and the x-ray equipment was so inadequate as to be highly dangerous to those operating it as well as to the patients. The Parish Council was persuaded, no doubt by the skilled advocacy of Dr Balfour Black, that a new department was essential. They were possibly equally convinced of the need for new equipment after considering its cost in comparison with the potential awards of damages to staff electrocuted in the execution of their duties. The Council therefore commissioned Colonel Donald J Mackintosh, medical superintendent of the Western Infirmary, to design an up-to-date department of radiology. The new department was opened formally in 1928. Two nursing sisters, neither of whom had much experience of radiography, were appointed to the department. Organised tuition was not available and Dr Balfour Black undertook their training. Both were successful in obtaining their MSR certificates and ultimately became superintendent radiographers.

In 1961 Sidney Haase came from the Royal Infirmary. The other consultants who joined the department were Agnes MacGregor, who came from the Southern General Hospital and Craigie Anton. John R M Wilson was appointed in 1967. Albert Aylmer worked in Stobhill for some time but was also radiologist at Knightswood Hospital and finally at Gartnavel General Hospital when it opened in 1973. On Sydney Haase's retiral Roy Sutherland became consultant in administrative charge and from 1987 to 1991 was in charge of both Stobhill and the Royal Infirmary. Joe Negrette was in day to day charge during this period and became head of department on Roy Sutherland's retiral. Bernard Anastasi was a consultant for a relatively short period before he left for a post in England. Joe Negrette subsequently left Stobhill for the Royal Alexandra Hospital, Paisley. He was replaced as lead consultant by Ian McLeod who had already been at Stobhill for some time. After a short time as consultant with an interest in interventional radiology Susan Ingram left for Edinburgh where her husband had been appointed consultant surgeon. The other consultants presently at Stobhill are John Shand, Fiona Bryden, Rhona Stevens, Gina McCreath and Michael Sproule. Gina McCreath had spent the greater part of her career at the Southern General Hospital before moving to Stobhill. Stobhill is the Glasgow centre for gynaecological malignancy. This has a large influence on its workload. Fiona Bryden has a particular interest in this and in thoracic radiology. A spiral CT scanner was installed in 1995.

Victoria Infirmary

The Victoria opened its first x-ray department in an extension built in 1902 (the present Ward 12). The very considerable expense of the installation, amounting to no less than £350, was met by Archibald Walker, a wealthy distiller and the Merchants' House representative on the board. The installation proved popular and for years the average daily attendance was about 20 patients. In 1912 it was reported that "x-rays and electrical treatment, no longer in its experimental stage, now forms an important part of the work of the infirmary… results have been very satisfactory". From the beginning, Duncan O MacGregor, the medical superintendent, had run the department himself and had thus gained much experience in the field of radiology. In 1919 he was formally appointed radiologist to the hospital, combining the duties with those of his administrative post. He was the sole radiologist.

Following his death in 1929 and until another appointment could be made, the work of the x-ray department was undertaken temporarily by the versatile surgeon, Robert Mailer, who had obtained some experience while at the Mayo Clinic. The vacancy was filled by the appointment of George Jackson Wilson, who until then had been radiologist at Stirling Royal Infirmary and Falkirk District Infirmary. Jackson Wilson graduated at Glasgow in 1911 and took the DPH, Cambridge in 1913. He served in the RAMC in France in the Great War. It was there that his interest in radiology was fostered. Soon after his appointment in 1929 the department was modernised and completely new equipment installed. With this Wilson provided a most efficient service but the ever increasing demands made on the department called for further extension. In this area his technical knowledge and planning ability were of great value although, because of his unassuming manner, this remained unknown to many. Jackson Wilson was also radiologist to the Royal Maternity Hospital for many years and continued in that capacity until 1955, nine years after his retiral from the Victoria. He died in 1961 at the age of 75.

John Innes was appointed successor to Jackson Wilson in 1946. He had the advantage of having been an engineer before he became a doctor. He graduated with a BSc in engineering and MB ChB in 1937, both from Aberdeen University. He became a resident radiological officer at the Christie Hospital and Holt Radium Institute in Manchester. With the qualification of DMRE, he returned to Aberdeen and was radiologist at Woodend Hospital and assistant radiologist at Aberdeen Royal Infirmary. His exceptional technical knowledge was invaluable in the developments which took place under his direction. In 1966 the new out-patient department was opened. X-ray facilities were provided in the accident and emergency department on the ground floor and a full angio-cardiographic facility was opened on the top floor. This was not an ideal location because of its distance from the main x-ray department and the inability of the small lifts designed for out-patients to take a bed and accompanying resuscitation equipment. Its use for cardiology ceased when cardiac surgery was transferred from Mearnskirk Hospital to the Royal Infirmary. It provided a useful facility for ERCPs as well as angiography until it was closed in 1997. Karel Blum was John Innes's colleague for many years and such was his personality that many people thought he was "chief". After his retiral in 1966 Dr Blum continued to be a well known figure in the west of Scotland. He continued doing locums into his 80s.

John Lawson joined the department in 1953 and Harry Gardner in 1961. Dr Lawson succeeded Dr Innes as head of department.

The most influential radiologist at the Victoria in recent memory is Stuart Davidson. A Glasgow graduate, he came to the Victoria from Dundee, where he had been a senior registrar. He was particularly interested in medical education and put a huge amount of work into establishing a film library which is still used extensively today by registrars throughout the west of Scotland. He succeeded John Lawson as chairman of the division of radiology in 1984 but sadly died at the age of 60 of pancreatic carcinoma shortly after demitting office in 1991. Dr Davidson had worked hard to persuade management to purchase a CT scanner but it was not installed till 1992. Even then, through the good offices of Alistair Mack, then medical director, it was largely funded by the Fraser Foundation. Dr Davidson is remembered in the Stuart Davidson Suite which was opened in 1997 by his widow and incorporates digital angiography, ultrasound and urology rooms.

He was succeeded by Mary Millar, who became a consultant in 1972, as chairman of division and subsequently clinical director. She retired in 1999. Stella Goudie was appointed to succeed John Lawson in 1984. She developed vascular and interventional radiology and had a particular interest in urological intervention until urology moved to the Southern General Hospital. George McInnes who spent a short time at the Victoria before leaving for Edinburgh, developed the interventional interest further. He was succeeded by Andrew Downie who came from Guy's and St. Thomas's in London. He has been very innovative in the further development of this service. John Calder, a former Victoria senior registrar came to the department from Aberdeen to succeed Harry Gardner in 1986. He succeeded Mary Millar as clinical director in 1997. He was President of the Scottish Radiological Society from 1997 to 1999 and, as such, took responsibility for writing this book.

After Stuart Davidson's death his post was split and expanded to incorporate breast screening which was becoming established at that time. These shared posts were taken up by Russell Pickard and Jean Lauder. Dr Pickard has continued in that capacity but Dr Lauder is now at the Victoria full-time, having taken over the cross sectional imaging from Graham McKillop who left for Edinburgh after only a short period.

The Southern General Hospital

The Southern General was opened as the Govan Poor House in 1872. Little has been recorded about early radiology there but it is known that the first x-ray department was formed when the core of the present department was converted from Ward 10. A Balfour Black was in charge of both the former Glasgow Corporation hospitals, the Southern General and Stobhill before 1960. Robert Crawford was also there and Agnes MacGregor and William Dempster were part-time SHMOs. They subsequently became consultants at Stobhill and Law Hospitals respectively.

John Knight Davidson was appointed consultant in administrative charge in 1960. At that time the Clyde Tunnel was nearing completion. Dr Davidson carried out an x-ray survey of tunnel workers in conjunction with the MRC Decompression Sickness Panel, and made this the subject of his MD thesis. His consultant colleagues were Wilson James and Kenneth Grossart who had a shared appointment with the Institute of Neurological Sciences. When "Jake" Davidson left for the Western Infirmary in 1967, Wilson James took charge. He was one of the first radiologists in Glasgow to take a serious interest in mammography and also organised the first Glasgow wide teaching programme in 1967. In 1971 a new wing was built and the Southern General installed the first simple working computer in an x-ray department in Scotland and possibly in the

United Kingdom and Europe. Dr James was joined by D A R (Sandy) Robertson in 1966 and Roy Sutherland in 1968. Both had trained in radiology in Edinburgh. In 1971 Gina McCreath, who had been a registrar and senior registrar in the Southern General, joined the team in 1978 two years after taking up her first consultant post at the Western Infirmary. Sandy Robertson succeeded Wilson James as consultant in administrative charge in 1987.

In 1997 the department was completely re-designed and enlarged and new equipment, including a helical CT scanner, was installed.

When Sandy Robertson retired in 1998 Grant Urquhart became clinical director. He and his colleague Robert Johnstone have a particular interest in vascular and interventional radiology. Both Colin Campbell and Paul Duffy have an interest in musculo-skeletal radiology. Dr Duffy has particular expertise in MRI although currently the only scanner available is at the Institute of Neurological Sciences. Louise Stewart, a former Southern General registrar left her first consultant post in Falkirk to join the department in 1998.

Institute of Neurological Sciences

The Institute started life in Killearn Hospital in 1966 when it was opened by Bruce Millan, Secretary of State for Scotland. The radiologists then were J Leslie Steven and Kenneth Grossart. Neuroradiological examinations at that time were restricted to plain films, Myodil myelography, lumbar air encephalography, ventriculography and angiography, the last three of which were usually carried out under general anaesthesia. The temporary war-time buildings at Killearn soon became inadequate and the Institute moved to its present site at the Southern General in 1970. Peter Macpherson joined the department at the time of the move. In 1973 the second commercially available EMI computed tomographic scanner was installed. This was a major advance but the early scanner gave little information about the pituitary, an area of special interest within the Institute. A modified combined ventriculogram/cisternogram performed by cisternal puncture was pioneered by Dr Macpherson in order to assess the suprasellar space. He also developed orbital venography to determine lateral spread of pituitary tumours into the cavernous sinus. These techniques have been supplanted by dynamic CT and MRI. CT in relationship to head injuries, in close association with the departments of neurosurgery and neuropathology, has been a major interest.

Myodil myelography has long since been supplanted by non ionic water-soluble myelography. This has in turn been almost completely replaced by MRI. During the 1970s percutaneous transfemoral angiography replaced direct puncture angiography under anaesthesia. The angiographic room has been replaced twice since 1970. The latest installation has a bi-plane digital subtraction unit. Dr Grossart pioneered peroperative angiography to ensure complete excision of cerebral arteriovenous malformations. Now arteriovenous malformations, intracranial aneurysms, carotico-cavernous fistulas and some tumours are treated by percutaneous angiographic techniques.

In 1984 a 0.15 Tesla MRI unit was installed with funding from an MRC grant. Donald Hadley, whose post was originally MRC funded, came from Aberdeen, the centre in Scotland where MRI had been pioneered. The resulting randomised trial investigating symptomatic posterior fossa lesions is the only one of its kind to assess the overall clinical impact of MRI compared with CT. In 1993 the low field scanner was replaced with a 1.5 Tesla MRI system which is capable of rapid multiplanar scanning, MR angiography and MR spectroscopy. However technology has progressed so rapidly that this machine is now urgently in need of replacement.

Following a successful research programme, based on a Welcome grant awarded jointly to the departments of clinical physics, neurosurgery and the neuroscientists in Glasgow University, into the use of single photon energy computed tomography in dementia, their dedicated nuclear medicine head scanner was rehoused in the department. It is now widely used to assess perfusion patterns associated with diseases such as epilepsy, stroke, and encephalitis and radionuclide uptake into tumours to assess their growth and adequacy of radiotherapy or resection in addition to receptor imaging in the selection of patients likely to respond to particular drugs.

As technology advanced, the workload varied. Digital images are now transferred for expert opinion from seven surrounding hospitals via the BT telephone system. As each new advance in imaging has developed it has been evaluated and then introduced into clinical practice usually replacing an older more invasive or more risky technique. One-fifth of the department's workload is now performed by MRI. In 1970 3,500 patients had relatively invasive examinations which carried a significant risk. In contrast in 1995 22,500 patients benefited from having generally non-invasive, low risk examinations.

Royal Hospital for Sick Children

In the early years of the hospital before 1916, it is recorded that on the upper floor of the dispensary worked the specialists — a dentist, an aurist, an oculist and, after Röntgen ray apparatus had been presented to the hospital, an honorary medical electrician. This may have been James Riddell who acted as a consultant to the Royal Hospital for Sick Children before he took up his appointment at the Western Infirmary.

In 1914 the hospital moved to its present site at Yorkhill. David Campbell Suttie was appointed to the new medical superintendent's post which he combined with the role of radiologist. His combined posts gave him the chance to assess the work of the surgeons. He could see their results on his x-ray plates — an early example of audit? Apart from the period of the Great War, when a layman was put in charge of x-rays, Suttie remained at the hospital till his retiral in 1953. By the mid 1930s, the old x-ray machine, once considered the best, was obsolete. In 1953 the posts of medical superintendent and radiologist were separated and Simon Philip Rawson was appointed radiologist. Dr Rawson's appointment marked the beginning of a more modern era in paediatric radiology but was unfortunately marred by his ill-health. His relatives donated the Rawson prize for the best paper given by a registrar.

Dr Rawson was joined by Elizabeth M Sweet who often had to take on the burden of running the department. In spite of this, she became one of Britain's leading paediatric radiologists, acknowledged when she became President of the European Society of Paediatric Radiologists and hosted its meeting in Glasgow in 1985.

The other radiologist in the early 1970s was Maimie McNair who had a shared post with the Western Infirmary. She left for King's College Hospital, London in 1977.

Mark Ziervogel, a South African who had trained in Glasgow, came to Yorkhill around 1978 after short spells as a consultant, firstly in New Zealand then in Falkirk. He had a particular interest in cranial neonatal ultrasound. He was for a time regional postgraduate education adviser and, in that capacity, was one of the first to point out the inadvisability of cutting radiology registrar numbers in the 1980s to "achieve a balance". That his advice and that of others was ignored by the management executive of the Scottish Office is evident in the current shortage of trained radiologists. When Elizabeth Sweet retired in 1988 Dr Ziervogel took over as head of department till he retired in 1992 at the early age of 56.

Ruth MacKenzie joined the department in 1979, originally in a shared post with the Western Infirmary. She has been head of department since 1992 and is the current clinical director. She has also had obstetric ultrasound sessions in Glasgow Royal Maternity Hospital. Her major interest is in nuclear medicine. The nuclear medicine department was set up in 1992, was expanded in 1996 and now has two gamma cameras running full-time. The department was one of the first in the world to write up the DMSA changes that occur in acute pyelonephritis and was the first in Scotland to use Krypton for lung scanning.

Anne Hollman joined the department in 1988 shortly after Elizabeth Sweet retired. She had a particular interest in ultrasound and had achieved national and international recognition. She gave lectures and tutorials on the subject in several countries. Sadly, her career was cut short when she died of bronchial adenocarcinoma on 27th November 1999.

In 1990 the first CT scanner was installed. Briony Fredericks came from Toronto Children's Hospital at this time because of her particular expertise in CT. The scanner, along with two gamma cameras, three ultrasound machines and the newly installed MRI scanner have all been charity funded. The other consultants recently appointed and currently in post are Alexander Maclennan and Sanjay Maroo, the first Kenyan to have been appointed as a consultant radiologist in Scotland.

Radiology in Public Health

Today there is much emphasis on screening programmes. Breast screening is well established and the extent of radiological involvement in a colo-rectal screening programme still has to be established. However, screening is not new as evidenced by the Glasgow x-ray campaign against tuberculosis.

Glasgow X-ray Campaign Against Tuberculosis

The campaign took place between 11th March and 12th April 1957.

In the years following the Second World War, Glasgow's record in tuberculosis had deteriorated until it had become the worst among British cities of a comparable size.

The introduction and extended use of mass radiography, the advent of BCG vaccination and the introduction of streptomycin in 1946 made control of tuberculosis a realistic possibility.

In September 1955 an approach was made to representatives of Glasgow Corporation by the Joint Under-Secretary of State (J Nixon Browne) and informal agreement to a city-wide mass radiography campaign was reached.

It was considered that five weeks was the longest period over which peak publicity could be sustained. It was accepted that each unit would be able to deal comfortably with 2,000 examinations per week. Previous experience in the United States and pilot studies undertaken in Scotland had indicated that the number which could be x-rayed per unit per day would be 350. The 10 Scottish mass miniature radiography units alone were considered unable to achieve these figures and substantial help was required from the remainder of the United Kingdom. Eventually 37 units in total were used in the campaign. With the exception of three units, all of the equipment was supplied by Messrs Watson Ltd who provided servicing throughout the period. The loss of time as a result of breakdowns was less than 3 per cent. In the event, the targets were greatly exceeded and on many occasions more than 2,000 examinations were carried out in one day by a unit. In the five weeks of the campaign 714,915 people (approximately 70% of the population) were x-rayed. The original target had been 420,000. A total of 2,842 active cases of tuberculosis and 5,370 cases requiring further observation was discovered.

The success of the campaign was due to meticulous planning, intensive publicity and public relations, the extremely hard work put in by paid and volunteer staff and by an unprecedented public response.

Breast Screening

Following the publication of the Forrest report on breast cancer screening in 1987, the first NHS funded Breast Screening Unit opened in the Woodside Place facility of the West of Scotland Breast Screening Service in May 1988. Over the next three years, five other centres were opened in Edinburgh, Dundee, Aberdeen, Irvine and Inverness. A second Glasgow centre opened in Govanhill in 1991.

Since its inception, the Scottish programme has adhered strictly to the Forrest recommendation; namely offering single view mammography to asymptomatic women aged 50–64 every three years. Women over the age of 64 can self refer. Recognising that each of these recommendations was based on scientific evidence at the time of the publication of the Forrest report, multi-centre UK trials were set up to review these recommendations. July 1995 saw the publication of data confirming that increased cancer detection could be achieved, with an associated reduction in the anxiety related to recall rate, by performing two views at prevalent attendance. This change in policy was taken on board. The publication of the trials examining optimal interval for screening and efficacy of screening in the 40–41 age group are awaited. The latest published figures for the Scottish programme reveal that the Pritchard published guidelines are being met in most criteria. In 1997/98: women invited 159,972, women attended 116,040 (72% of those invited); percentage of attenders recalled 11, cancers detected 4.6/1000 prevalent attenders and 4.0/1000 incident attenders.

The West of Scotland Breast Screening Service has recently completed a pilot project investigating the implications for the region should the age of attendance be extended to 69. The clinical director, Hilary Dobson, who has been in post since 1988, leads a team of eight mainly sessional radiologists dedicated to the screening programme.

Radiotherapy and Oncology

The Glasgow Cancer and Skin Institute was established at 400 St Vincent Street in 1886. Following a successful appeal for funds, a small house containing 10 beds was opened at 163 Hill Street, Garnethill under the directorship of Hugh Murray. He did not believe in the surgical treatment of cancer, a view at variance with that of many of his contemporaries. Following Murray's resignation in 1893 the Glasgow Cancer Hospital was established as a separate entity in 1894. A separate outpatient dispensary was opened at 22 West Graham Street and an outdoor nursing department was established for visiting and assisting cancer patients in their own homes. George (later Sir George) Beatson, a surgeon, was its first director. He recorded that between 1894 and 1922, the hospital treated 3,195 inpatients (1,225 males and 1,970 females) and looked after 1,128 outpatients (189 males and 939 females) in their own homes. The number of admissions rose from 84 in 1894 to 259 in 1922. Beatson's reputation rests on his demonstration of the effectiveness of oophorectomy in the treatment of some cases of breast cancer.

In 1912 a new 50 bed extension was opened by Princess Louise, Duchess of Argyll. It was granted the title of Glasgow Royal Cancer Hospital by King George V.

X-rays were used for treating cancer from the early days of medical electricity and Beatson published a paper in the British Medical Journal in 1902 on their use in the Glasgow Cancer Hospital. With the increasing use of x-rays, large departments for the treatment of cancer grew in Glasgow, mainly at the Royal and Western Infirmaries but also at the Victoria Infirmary, Stobhill Hospital and the Samaritan Hospital.

The Glasgow Cancer Hospital opened a research department early in its existence. Sir George Beatson was one of its first three directors. W E Walker was the first director of the research laboratory and (Sir) Harold Whittingham (later Air Marshall) its first pathologist. Their early work was concerned with the morphology of chromosomes and aberrations occurring in cancer cells.

In 1928 Lady Burrell made a gift of £10,000 for the purchase of half a gram of radium.

Following visits to the Middlesex Hospital and the Curie Foundation in Paris, Dr Peacock, Dr Walker's successor as director, established the Radium Institute. It agreed to lend radium to other institutions provided they agreed to a uniform plan of treatment, record keeping and statistical publication.

The Royal and Victoria Infirmaries, the Ear Nose and Throat Hospital and hospitals at Paisley and Greenock agreed to this proposal but the Western Infirmary wished to keep its own store of radium.

The speciality of radiotherapy gradually developed between 1920 and 1940 and, soon after the Second World War, megavoltage x– and gamma rays came into use. This was helped by two by-products of wartime research — the linear accelerator (which used radar technique) and the telecobalt unit (using radioactive cobalt from a nuclear reactor). The size, cost and complexity of these machines meant that rationalisation of radiotherapy services was inevitable. The separation of diagnostic radiology from radiotherapy and the establishment of the National Health Service in 1948 were further stimuli for change. After 1948 the emphasis on cancer at the Glasgow Royal Cancer Hospital was reduced by the introduction of departments of urology and general surgery. In 1952 the hospital was renamed the Royal Beatson Memorial Hospital.

In 1966 the Glasgow Institute of Radiotherapeutics and Oncology was established by the amalgamation of the units at the Western and Royal Infirmaries with the Royal Beatson Memorial Hospital. A new department was set up at Belvidere Hospital to replace that at the Royal. Keith Halnan was the first director and was subsequently succeeded by Gerald Flatman then Thurston Brewin. In 1966 the institute had 128 beds in two main treatment departments, the Western and Belvidere. In 1967 the research department strengthened its independent status and acquired the name of The Beatson Institute for Cancer Research. Its continued expansion led to a move to its present site on Garscube Estate in 1976.

In 1974 (Sir) Kenneth Calman was appointed as the first Professor of Clinical Oncology. He subsequently became Dean of Postgraduate Medicine at Glasgow University, Chief Medical Officer of Scotland, then of England. He is now Vice Chancellor of Durham University. He was succeeded by Stanley Kaye. The first Professor of Radiation Oncology is Ann Barrett who was appointed in 1986.

In 1988 the department of medical oncology was amalgamated with the department of radiotherapy at the Western Infirmary with Ann Barrett as its director. It then merged with the department at Belvidere Hospital and was renamed the Beatson Oncology Centre. The Royal Beatson Memorial Hospital closed in 1989 and at that time the Cancer Research Campaign donated about £800,000 to enable a new ward for the medical oncologists and suite of offices to be opened. The altered unit was opened by Sir Alexander Currie, then Director of the Cancer Research Campaign. Belvidere Hospital closed in 1996 by which time two new units had been installed at the Beatson Oncology Centre, Western Infirmary. In 1998 Sam Galbraith, then Scottish Minister for Health, announced that the Scottish Office was giving £9.9 million to allow the Beatson to build phase one at Gartnavel General Hospital. This will have five bunkers, with three new treatment machines, one or two of which will be replacements. There will also be a small out patient facility. Work started on 1st November 1999.

The Beatson Oncology Centre is now the second largest of its kind in Britain. Its aims are similar to those of the first Glasgow cancer hospital: to provide the best possible treatment and care for patients with cancer; to educate all involved in that care to the highest standard; by means of research, both clinical and laboratory, to improve understanding and treatment of cancer.

3

Edinburgh

Royal Infirmary

In 1898 the Infirmary's first electrical department was opened in cramped quarters in a former paint store and plumber's workshop. In 1904 the department moved to larger premises but, by 1920 extension of the use of x-rays from diagnosis to therapy of cancer and other conditions meant that the equipment and accommodation were no longer adequate.

The first medical electrician was Dawson Turner whose biographical details are written in the opening chapter. He was joined in 1901 by William Hope Fowler and later by Archibald McKendrick. A reply from McKendrick to a letter from George Pirie of Dundee is illustrative of the workload of the time:

"Dear Sir,
I have your kind enquiry re our routine in x-ray Dept. Of Royal Infirmary.
Our work has increased and we now do about 6000 radiographs annually.
These we index according to the name of the patient, region, disease etc. What I suppose you would wish however is a way out of you own difficulty. You do not say if you have any help at all. Dr Hope Fowler and I are jointly in charge of the Medical Electrical Dept. This includes all forms of electrical treatment — a large separate Balneological Dept. and X-Ray work. Our assistants are as follows.
1 Nurse who attends to galvanic and faradic methods of treatment only.
I Boy who develops plates and keeps instruments clean. (about 20/- per week.) This boy is supervised by our mechanic in the

Dept. about 12 years (salary £100 per year). He takes x-rays
— keeps tubes in order — goes over every tube every morning
and records its condition as to hardness etc.
Then we have a qualified Clinical Assistant who helps Dr Fowler
and myself (honorarium £25 annually).
Dr Hope Fowler has an honorarium of £100 per annum. I
have an honorarium of £75 per an. To be raised to £100 two
years hence.
If this is not exactly the information you are after do not
hesitate to write.
Yours faithfully,
Archd. M Kendrick
Dr Fowler is off with influenza just now."

Like Dawson Turner, Hope Fowler did not escape the effects of
repeated exposure to x-rays and eventually died in 1933, a martyr
to radiology.

In 1914 consideration had been given to providing a new
building but plans were inevitably abandoned on the outbreak
of war. In 1923 a special committee of the board was appointed
under the convenership of Sir James Hodsdon and a site selected for
the new building. The building was designed by Thomas Turnbull
with advice from Robert Knox, radiologist from King's College
Hospital, London, to meet the requirements of J Woodburn
Morison, the infirmary's radiologist. It was situated on unoccupied
ground between the surgical and medical houses, contiguous
with a long corridor and balcony which connected it to both
houses. As the dangers of exposure to x-rays had become
recognised, great care had been taken to ensure adequate radiation
protection. To ensure the safety of operators and others in the
new building, exhaustive experiments were undertaken as a
result of which the walls were constructed of concrete slabs into
which barium sulphate had been introduced in the proportion
found to give the highest level of protection combined with
sufficient strength. The walls were also coated on both sides with
barium plaster. The basement contained the heavy electrical
machinery, the mechanics' work shops, the stores and the safe for
radium. The ground floor accommodated the apparatus for x-
ray diagnosis and therapy, the dark rooms and a large room for
the purposes of demonstration and teaching. The cost of

construction including part of the fittings and equipment was £39,500. An additional sum of £9,087 was required for installation of the x-ray plant, bringing the total to £48,587. The cost was met in part by a gift of £15,000 from the City of Edinburgh branch of the British Red Cross Society and in part from a special appeal. The official opening ceremony was performed on 9th October 1926 by the Duke of York.

In June 1923 the managers of the Royal Infirmary suggested to the University Court that it should consider the institution of a lectureship in medical therapeutics and radiology. The court agreed on the understanding that the university should have an adequate voice in the selection of the person whom the managers might appoint in charge of the department. In 1924 the board appointed John Miller Woodburn Morison, the head of the radiological department. In 1925 the university appointed Morison lecturer in radiology and contributed £400 towards his salary on condition that the equipment of the department should be available for the instruction of students without further charge (to the university). In 1926 the University Court established a diploma in radiology.

Morison resigned in 1930 and was replaced by J Duncan White who, in turn, left in 1934 to return to London. His successor, Alfred E Barclay, came from Cambridge but he was dogged by ill-health and had to resign in 1934. However, on his appointment, Barclay had been accompanied by a senior assistant radiologist, Robert McWhirter, who succeeded him as head of department at the age of 31.

Robert McWhirter was born in Ballantrae in 1904. He graduated in medicine with high commendation from the University of Glasgow in 1927. He trained in radiology in Cambridge, London and the Mayo Clinic and subsequently accepted a research fellowship with Ralston Peterson at the Christie Hospital in Manchester.

The accommodation and equipment which he inherited in Edinburgh were, in his own words, more suitable for a museum than for use in a hospital. Each time an x-ray was taken, the room was filled with stray radiation and, in the damp atmosphere of Edinburgh, frequently threw an arc of lightning across the gap, with a loud crack of thunder. Soon after his appointment, he submitted a comprehensive report on the department with plans for its improvement. Whereas Duncan White, on leaving the department in 1934, had suggested that a sum of £500 would bring the department up to date, McWhirter recommended that all the old apparatus in the department was either out of date or useless and should be replaced by modern apparatus. The managers accepted his recommendations and four years later, reported that the work had been completed at a cost of £14,500 for equipment (including £5,000 for Metropolitan-Vickers apparatus introduced by Barclay) and £7,660 for reconstruction. Staffing levels had also been greatly increased. In 1946 McWhirter was appointed to the newly endowed Forbes Chair of Medical Radiology in the University of Edinburgh, a post which he held till his retirement in 1970. Soon after this appointment, he decided that diagnostic radiology and radiotherapy should be separated. The rest of his work will be considered in the section on radiotherapy and oncology.

Before the departments separated, John Paton McGibbon was appointed senior assistant radiologist in 1942. He was born in 1904, son of a professor of midwifery. Following poliomyelitis in childhood, he recovered sufficiently to win the junior 100 yards at Edinburgh Academy but at 16 he contracted diphtheria and scarlet fever which were to leave him severely handicapped by extensive dorsal scoliosis and atrophy of both legs. Despite these handicaps, further aggravated by severe migraine, he graduated MB ChB at Edinburgh University in 1929. He originally studied infectious diseases, taking his DPH in 1932 and was awarded an MD in 1933 for a thesis on "The Cutaneous Reactions to Products of the Haemolytic Streptococcus in Scarlet Fever and Erysipelas and the Anomalies of the Dick Test".

Dr McGibbon's frail health induced him to change careers from clinical medicine to radiology and he obtained his diploma in 1935. After a period as assistant radiologist at the Western Infirmary, Glasgow, he returned to the Royal where he made himself a master in his chosen field. His advice on difficult problems was frequently sought and his opinion highly respected by his fellow radiologists and by the clinicians of the hospital. He contributed in a large measure to the advances which took place in Edinburgh and in particular, was a pioneer of cardiac radiology. It is, however, as a clinical teacher that he is best remembered. He had the rare gift of patience and an unusual ability to appreciate the difficulties of his students. Many radiologists both British and from overseas, benefited from his skill and scrupulous care.

John McGibbon died following an accident in 1952. He is remembered by an annual eponymous lecture of the Scottish Radiological Society.

Separation of the departments of diagnostic and therapeutic radiology gave rise to 10 difficult years when they had to work together in the same area as had been used for the combined department. This problem was not solved till the radiotherapy department moved to the Western General Hospital in 1957. In addition, the number of diagnostic examinations increased from 42,000 in 1947 to 76,000 in 1957. The complexity of many of the examinations also increased. 2,000 of these examinations were carried out in outlying units including the Simpson Pavilion and around 50,000 in the department itself. The work done centrally represented (on the basis of a six-day week), the use of about 500 films daily or around one film every twenty seconds at peak periods. This was compounded by the 30 minutes required to develop each film before the introduction of automatic processors. The problem of containing the work increased year by year.

In 1945 William S Shearer joined the department as an assistant radiologist. An Edinburgh graduate, he had practised radiology in Manchester for eight years and had served as specialist radiologist during the Second World War, mainly in the Middle East. He was appointed director of the new radio-diagnostic department and continued in post for its first 10 difficult years. Sadly, before he was able to benefit from the new arrangements, Dr Shearer died suddenly in 1957. After an interim year when D W Lindsay was in charge, Eric Samuel was appointed director.

Eric Samuel was born in South Wales in 1914. He commenced his medical training in Cardiff and completed it in the Middlesex Hospital, graduating with honours in 1936. He took his FRCS in 1937, graduated MD in London in 1939, obtained his DMRE at Cambridge and became a fellow of the Royal College of Radiologists in 1941. Following military service in the Second World War his work on war wounds earned him the Röntgen award of the British Institute of Radiology. In 1946 he was the youngest ever honorary consultant to be appointed at the Middlesex Hospital. In 1947 he went to Pretoria, South Africa, where he stayed till he was appointed director of radiology at the Royal Infirmary in 1958. Eric Samuel became one of Scotland's foremost radiologists and his reputation and influence spread well beyond Edinburgh. His achievements at the Royal included the re-organisation of the department, the setting up of an intensive training programme for radiologists and the development of newer techniques such as angiography, operative cholangiography and mammography. A graph prepared by Samuel for the period 1930 to 1963 showed that the total number of patients admitted to the Infirmary had risen from 20,000 to 27,000 (an increase of 35%) while over the same period, the number of radiological examinations had increased from 15,000 to 100,000 (an increase of 556%).

In 1963 the department of medicine moved to a new building, enabling radiology to extend into its present accommodation. This helped deal with the rapidly developing advances in the speciality. These included the development of angiocardiography in 1966/67, ultrasound, nuclear medicine and, ultimately CT (the first whole body scanner in 1979) and MRI.

When Robert McWhirter retired in 1970, Eric Samuel was appointed to the Forbes Chair of Medical Radiology and a new chair of radiotherapy was created by the University. When Prof Samuel retired to South Africa in 1978, he had accumulated many honours and distinctions, including appointments as Hunterian Professor of the Royal College of Surgeons of England (1956), Knox Lecturer (1968) and Glyn Evans Lecturer (1974) in the Faculty of Radiologists, Scott Heron Lecturer to the University of Belfast (1969) and visiting professorships at Stanford University and the University of Pennsylvania. He was also Vice President of the Faculty of Radiologists (19616–2) and Treasurer (1962–68).

The relationship between McWhirter and Samuel was not always an easy one and it is said that in 1959 McWhirter had chosen five trainees in radiology. These were rejected by Samuel who chose five of his own, including Bruce Young and Ronald Mahaffy, later a consultant in Aberdeen.

In 1978 Prof Samuel was succeeded as Forbes Professor by Jonathan Best, an Edinburgh graduate who had trained in

Manchester. He was succeeded as consultant in administrative charge by Thomas Philp.

Tom Philp had been a consultant in the department since 1956. He had taken an interest in cardiovascular radiology at a time of rapid evolution and had a great commitment to teaching. In 1971 he was elected to a World Health Organisation Travelling Fellowship which took him to Japan, from where he returned full of enthusiasm for new developments in gastrointestinal radiology. He was Treasurer of the Royal College of Radiologists from 1983 to 1988 and President of the Scottish Radiological Society from 1978 to 1979. He retired in 1986 following a myocardial infarct. His retirement is commemorated by an annual award for the best original work by an Edinburgh junior radiologist. Alastair Kirkpatrick succeeded him as head of department.

Other consultant radiologists at the Royal during Eric Samuel's and Tom Philp's periods in charge included Michael Summerling, Tony Donaldson (a neuroradiologist of whom more will be said later) and James Duncan who later became consultant in administrative charge at Glasgow Royal Infirmary. Bruce Young was the first Edinburgh radiologist to provide an obstetric ultrasound service at the Simpson Pavilion, firstly with a Kretz A and B scanner in 1969 then with a Diasonograph in 1971. Michael Summerling became one of the first to use a Diasonograph at the Royal. He left for Newcastle when he failed to be appointed to the chair on Eric Samuel's retiral.

One of the most influential radiologists at the Royal Infirmary was T A S (Mike) Buist, a pioneer of interventional techniques. An Edinburgh graduate, he spent his national service with the Royal Airforce Mountain Rescue Service, then spent some time in general practice before training in radiology. He spent a year as a staff radiologist at Toronto General Hospital where his interest in vascular investigative procedures was stimulated. He was appointed consultant and part-time senior lecturer in 1969. He was one of the leading radiologists in the United Kingdom in the development of modern angiographic and interventional techniques. He became a member of the Interventional Radiology Group of the Royal College of Radiologists in 1982. Only weeks before his untimely death from gastric carcinoma in 1985 he addressed a meeting of the Royal College of Radiologists in Aberdeen.

Mike Buist has left a strong legacy in vascular and interventional radiology which has been taken forward by Doris Redhead, John Reid (before he left for Borders District General Hospital), Ian Gillespie, Kieron McBride, George McInnes and Susan Ingram.

In 1999 Tim Buckenham, who has a particular interventional interest, was appointed professor.

Musculo-skeletal radiology, including MRI, has been developed by Ian Beggs (clinical director until 2000) and by Irene Prossor.

Eric Samuel's and Bruce Young's early work on mammography has been taken forward into the era of breast screening by Alastair Kirkpatrick, Nicé Muir and James Walsh. Obstetric ultrasound is done by Jane Walker, one of the few radiologists in Scotland to have this interest.

Paul Allan is well known in the field of ultrasound. He is currently President of the British Medical Ultrasound Society and, with Grant Baxter of Glasgow, has just published a textbook on the subject.

Graham McKillop came from Glasgow in 1997 to take the major interest in CT and MRI.

Western General Hospital

In 1947 Hunter Cummack was appointed as consultant radiologist to the Edinburgh Corporation Hospitals, based at the Western General. He retained those posts at the inception of the National Health Service in 1948.

Hunter Cummack was born in 1914 in Kirkgunzeon in Kirkcudbrightshire. He was educated at Dumfries Academy and graduated MB ChB from Edinburgh University in 1936. After a brief period in general practice, he trained in radiology in Edinburgh. He obtained the FRCS (Ed) in 1939, the DMRD in 1940 and the FFR (RCSI) in the same year. In the Second World War, he was one of the officers appointed to guard Rudolf Hess on whom he performed a cholecystogram. Later he served in North Africa and in Italy where he was mentioned in dispatches.

On taking up his post at the Western General after the war, Dr Cummack developed a particular interest in gastro-intestinal radiology. His meticulous technique for barium meals and enemas was probably unrivalled at the time, bearing in mind that there was no image intensification and the procedure required a lengthy period of dark adaptation with goggles. He used the wealth of clinical material which he had collected to publish "Gastrointestinal X-Ray Diagnosis: A Descriptive Atlas" in 1969. In 1974 he was elected President of the Scottish Radiological Society and through negotiations with the Faculty (from 1975 Royal College) of Radiologists, was instrumental in setting up the Standing Scottish Committee. In recognition of his services, he was awarded the FRCR without examination. He retired in 1977 and died in 1996 at the age of 81.

In 1948 the x-ray department was a room off the main hospital corridor. The single room had two tables, one horizontal, the other erect. The patient had to be moved from one to the other if erect and supine films were required. The dark room had no ventilation. The film processor was made by a local joiner. The films were dried by hanging them from a washing line attached to the ceiling. There were two mobile units, one of which was United States army surplus stock. There was a waiting room for patients, part of which was screened off with a mobile screen. This served as the radiologist's office and reporting room. Patients who had had barium examinations were requested to go to a toilet down the corridor. When Cummack asked for toilet facilities for these patients he was advised by hospital board officials that patients should use a bucket in the x-ray room.

In 1955 Norman Thomson took over the Eastern General and City hospitals from Hunter Cummack. William A Copland was appointed in 1956 to cover the radiotherapy diagnostic work at the Northern General Hospital and the increasing volume of work at the Western. In 1957 radiotherapy moved from the Royal Infirmary to the Western General, increasing the need for supporting diagnostic services. In succeeding years, the department continued to grow in size. In 1971 the main department moved to new premises with 16 rooms in phase one. This was later expanded to 24 rooms.

In 1973 D J (Danny) Sinclair who later moved to Dundee, initiated an ultrasound service and was also responsible for isotope scanning. Ultrasound was carried on and expanded by Roger Wild who has become nationally known in the field. He became clinical director in 1992. Following Hunter Cummack's retiral in 1977, Martin Fraser took over as head of department and also continued to provide the gastrointestinal service. He made an extensive contribution to the literature on double contrast radiology. Gastrointestinal investigation was further progressed into ERCP by John Cruikshank and Douglas Grieve. Grieve has also made a major contribution to interventional radiology, particularly in renal and splenic embolisation, renal angioplasty and biliary drainage procedures. One of Scotland's first helical CT scanners was purchased in 1992, its speed of scanning being very useful in the large numbers of examinations emanating from the department of clinical oncology and haematology.

Colin Turnbull, the current clinical director, is a leader in the field of cardiac radiology. With Dr T R D Shaw, he performed the first mitral balloon valvuloplasty. In 2000 he took over as first Patient Services Director of the new Lothians University Hospitals NHS Trust, incorporating the Royal Infirmary, the Western General Hospital and the Royal Hospital for Sick Children.

Nuclear Medicine

The Western General is one of only two hospitals in Scotland recognised for training in nuclear medicine. The other is Glasgow Royal Infirmary. It is unique in that the service has been developed and lead by a radiologist. Malcolm Merrick came to the Western in 1974 after training in radiology and specifically in nuclear medicine in Oxford, Northwick Park and the Hammersmith Hospital. Nuclear medicine in Edinburgh had originally been set up by John Strong, professor of medicine at the Western, who had been involved in the radio-immuno assay of hormones and in the use of radioisotopes both diagnostically and therapeutically, but without imaging. John Strong had been instrumental in the creation of Malcolm Merrick's post. This post carried three university sessions as part-time senior lecturer. Some early work had also been carried out by Tony Donaldson at the department of surgical neurology, using a rectilinear scanner. Danny Sinclair had been responsible for isotope scanning at the Western and at the Royal Edinburgh Hospital for Sick Children before 1974.

In 1973 nuclear medicine was revolutionised by the advent of the Ohio Nuclear Gamma camera. Malcolm Merrick was able to obtain one of these cameras in 1975 at a cost of £50,000. The following year he obtained approval to purchase and interface a mini-computer. This improved the quality of low-count images and renal work. As the workload developed, two trends became apparent, namely the increasing number of requests for bone scans and the large number of patients referred from the Borders, Fife and the Lothians. A Cleon multi-detector scanner was purchased to cope with this load. After six years' service, the bolts holding the upper head assembly weighing over 100 kg failed and it crashed on to the couch which had just been vacated by a patient. That was the end of the Cleon but by good luck, no-one was killed or injured. A mobile service was eventually instituted for the hospitals in South East Scotland, using an Elscint Dymax camera. This service ran for almost 10 years till 1988, when it became too unreliable and the hospitals visited acquired their own gamma cameras. In its working life, it had covered over 80,000 miles and had performed almost 20,000 examinations.

The department, under Malcolm Merrick's guidance, has carried out research in several fields including bone scintigraphy, the role of bile-acids in malabsorption and renal investigations, particularly in children. Merrick, Uttley and Wild published two of the first papers on the role of isotope imaging techniques in the management of children with urinary tract infection. These are still quoted although superseded by the much larger and longer study by Merrick, Uttley, Notghi and Wilkinson in "Archives of Disease in Childhood" in 1995. In 1981 Merrick was approached to write a textbook of nuclear medicine. "The Essentials of Nuclear Medicine" was published in 1984, then completely re-written and re-published by Springer in 1997. Malcolm Merrick retired in 1999 and has been replaced by Martin Errington, a former Edinburgh registrar.

Department of Clinical Neurosciences

The building of the department of surgical neurology at the Western General in the late 1950s provided the opportunity to plan and equip a neuroradiological department serving the whole of South East Scotland and beyond. The neuroradiologist associated with this project was Andrew Alexander (Tony) Donaldson who was one of the pioneers of neuroradiology in the United Kingdom.

Tony Donaldson was born and educated in Edinburgh and qualified LRCP (Ed), LRFP&S (Glas) in 1945. Even before his National Service in the Royal Navy, he had come under the influence of the noted neurosurgeon, Norman Dott. On his return to civilian life Tony was appointed neurosurgical registrar at the Royal Infirmary. After several years of pursuing a neurosurgical career he was persuaded to undertake radiological training and obtained the DMRD (Ed) in 1953. He was immediately appointed senior registrar then consultant in 1956. Over the years he held this post, he continued to develop and modernise the department, introducing new apparatus and techniques. Many of these were superseded by computed tomography and later by MRI. One of the first CT scanners in Scotland was installed in the department in 1973.

Tony Donaldson was widely recognised as a clinical teacher and trainees from many countries were attracted to his department. Throughout his career he published widely and lectured to radiological meetings and congresses throughout the world. His contribution to neuroradiology was recognised by his election to the fellowships of the Royal Colleges of Physicians and of Surgeons of Edinburgh and of the Royal College of Radiologists. He became President of the Scottish Radiological Society and the British Society of Neuroradiologists. He died suddenly while playing golf at Gleneagles on 17th May 1987.

The work of the department has been carried forward by a team of neuroradiologists, including George Vaughan, Robin Sellar, Joanna Wardlaw and Roderick Gibson. Interventional techniques have progressed rapidly, particularly in relation to the treatment of arterio-venous malformations with glue and particles, carotico-cavernous fistulas with balloons and aneurysms with coils. CT and, increasingly MRI, provide the mainstay of the department's work.

The Royal Edinburgh Hospital for Sick Children

In 1897 two years after the opening of the present hospital, a department of medical electricity was opened with Harry Rainy as medical electrician. John Spence, who had been Dawson Turner's assistant at the Royal Infirmary since 1901, succeeded Rainy in 1907. The potential and indeed the risks of x-rays had not been appreciated fully and Spence became one of the x-ray martyrs. However, he served the hospital well for 22 years, from his appointment till he retired in 1929. In 1914 it is recorded that he took 1,004 "skiagrams". Not only was he well versed in the work of the new speciality but also his keen sense of humour endeared him to the children. His appearances as Father Christmas at annual parties were memorable.

In 1929 Dr Spence was succeeded by Grant Allan who retired in 1956 after 27 years' service. From 1947 to 1976 William McLeod held a joint appointment with the Deaconess Hospital.

Danny Sinclair had a shared consultant post with the Western General Hospital from 1972 to 1975. He was responsible for introducing the concept of renal isotope scanning to William Uttley, one of the paediatricians. Both Danny Sinclair and Roger Wild, who succeeded him in the shared post in 1975, were important figures in the development of ultrasound. Dr Sinclair became a consultant in Dundee and Dr Wild gave up his paediatric sessions in 1986 to go full-time at the Western General.

The present head of department, Michael Hendry took up a shared appointment with the Deaconess Hospital in 1977 and dropped his sessions at the latter in 1983 to devote all of his time to the Sick Children's. He was joined by Stephanie Mackenzie in 1986, Maeve McPhillips in 1995 and Graham Wilkinson in 1998.

At the time of writing the hospital has just installed its first MRI scanner.

Other Edinburgh Hospitals

Since 1st April 1999 the other hospitals in Edinburgh and East Lothian have merged with primary care to form the Lothian Primary Care Trust. The hospitals which have been incorporated in the new trust are the Eastern General Hospital, Liberton Hospital, Edenhall in Musselburgh, Roodlands in Haddington, Leith Hospital, The Royal Edinburgh and Astley Ainsley Hospitals. As so many hospitals, some of them small, are involved, history is fragmented and not well recorded. Some of the hospitals in the group were the responsibility of Edinburgh Corporation until the inception of the National Health Service.

From 1947 Hunter Cummack, based at the Western General Hospital, was also consultant radiologist to the Northern General, Eastern General, City Hospital and Gogarburn.

It is known that Leith Hospital installed x-ray equipment in 1904 and that this was seen as an opportunity to raise much needed money. Appropriate cases of malignant disease were being treated with radium in the 1930s under the care of the lady superintendent. In 1942 Robert McWhirter was appointed consulting radiologist/radiotherapist with a view to organising cancer treatment on an area basis.

In 1978 Martin Fraser, who had had sessions at the hospital, left to become full-time radiologist at the Western General. He was succeeded by Douglas Grieve who also had the majority of his sessions at the Western General and is now there full time. In 1986 a small three-roomed department with one part-time radiologist had 12,261 patient attendances, including 890 contrast and 463 ultrasound examinations. From August 1987 it served outpatient clinics and general practitioner referrals only. At the time, it was the only hospital in Edinburgh to offer a full range of examinations to direct general practitioner access. Leith Hospital is temporarily closed for refurbishment and, when it re-opens, will provide imaging for the new Primary Care Trust.

Before a previous re-organisation in 1986/87 the Eastern General and Edenhall Hospitals stood alone, following a breakdown in relations in the old north sector. They were staffed by one consultant and 0.4 senior registrar sessions till the latter were withdrawn on educational grounds. When the east unit was formed in 1987 it included the Eastern General, Edenhall, Leith, Roodlands and East Fortune (now closed). In 1987 H L (Lind) McDonald was appointed consultant to replace Norman Thomson. At the time there were 1.9 whole time equivalent consultants, including 4 sessions at Leith and a shared post with Western General held by Douglas Grieve. Norman Speirs held a split post between the Royal Edinburgh Hospital and Roodlands.

In October 1987 a second full-time post was established at the Eastern General and Edenhall Hospitals and filled by Richard Adam. Norman Speirs retired and was replaced by Alan Stevenson who held a post evenly split between the Eastern and Western General Hospitals. In 1990 he gave up his Eastern commitment in favour of the Western General. Lind McDonald and Richard Adam took up the Roodlands sessions. Jane Walker joined the establishment as consultant in 1995 but later left for the Royal Infirmary and Simpson Pavilion. Sarah Chambers moved in the opposite direction to replace her. Prof Jonathan Best, still employed by the University of Edinburgh, is the radiologist at the Royal Edinburgh and Astley Ainsley hospitals.

West Lothian

Bangour Hospital was built as an asylum in 1904 and became a military hospital in the First World War. The original asylum had an x-ray department and this was expanded during the war under the charge of Mr Thomas Rankine. The department had three rooms which was a more generous allocation of space than that afforded to most of the major hospitals in the country at the time. An x-ray machine, gifted by the American Red Cross, was described as having a 10 horsepower motor and a dynamo capable of delivering 15 KVA energy at the tube, a closed arc transformer with five steps of transformation from 25,000 to 100,000 volts, and a special arrangement for fluoroscopy, a trolley switchboard and an automatic time switch. It was selected after a trial of seven other machines. It delivered with ease 100 to 150 milliamperes at the tube and enabled exposures to be made in a fraction of a second or less. The tubes were almost all of American manufacture, Macalister Wiggin, Bauer and Coolidge.

By 1947 the staff consisted of a visiting radiologist, Robert Saffley, three radiographers and one student. In 1948 10,000 patients were examined. In the 1940s and early 1950s, much of the radiographic work was in pulmonary and spinal tuberculosis. Prof Norman Dott had beds at Bangour and generally the only calls for x-rays out of working hours were from his unit. In 1968 the total number of patients examined had risen to 26,000. Kenneth Wood was appointed consultant at that time to help cope with the increasing workload. In 1969 a casualty department opened and a full on call/standby radiographic service was introduced. It was kept very busy by the nearby Edinburgh to Glasgow road which had one of the highest accident rates in Britain. Robert Saffley retired in 1974 and was replaced by Alastair McKintosh who left in 1983. Andrew Duncan had a short appointment between 1979 and 1980. Ian Parker was appointed in 1981 and Peta S V Reddy in 1983. As the result of the hard work and dedication of Ian Parker, a computer software system to run a patient record system was devised. This speeded up the reporting time of x-rays and kept figures for annual statistical returns.

In 1991 the department moved to the new hospital of St. John's at Howden and had the advantage of being re-equipped from the start. Much of this equipment is now due for replacement but, due in no small part to Ian Parker's business skills, provision for this has been made. Following the expansion in work generated by the move to new premises, additional radiologists were required. Lesley Smart was appointed in 1993, Melanie Chapman had a short stay from 1994 to 1996, Peter Bailey was appointed in 1997, Tom Fitzgerald in 1997 and Carolyn Beveridge in 1999. Peta Reddy retired in 1997. Ian Parker remains in administrative charge.

The Borders

Radiological services in the borders were originally provided at Peel Hospital, Galashiels. Sam McCall Smith came from Dumfries as radiologist in 1972 and was joined by Iain Houston in 1976. Dr McCall-Smith retired in 1982 and was replaced by David Hardwick in 1984.

The new Borders General Hospital was opened in Melrose in 1988. Andrew Pearson was appointed at that time and since then has been joined by Hamish McRitchie, John Reid and Helen Shannon in a modern department, which includes a CT scanner and a gamma camera, and provides a comprehensive radiological service for the Borders.

Breast Screening

The breast screening programme came about through the production of the report on breast cancer commissioned by the Department of Health, under the leadership of Patrick Forrest, the Regius Professor of Surgery in Edinburgh. The report was commissioned in 1985 and completed in 1987, with a recommendation that a nationwide breast cancer screening programme would be able to reduce the mortality rate from breast cancer in the population.

In Scotland, the programme was set up in essentially the same way as in England and Wales but there were a few significant differences. Each health department established a national advisory group to advise the Management Executive in Scotland and in England respectively on the establishment and running of the programme. In Scotland, Alastair Kirkpatrick was able to use his place on the national advisory group to persuade it to recommend to the National Executive that double film reading by two radiologists would be advisable to maximise the sensitivity of the mammographic screening test. This was implemented. South of the border this was not the case and reliance was placed officially on single reading, although at least half the English screening programmes are managing unofficially to carry out double reading. It has been shown that double reading has resulted in an average gain of 10% in the number of cancers detected by the programme in Scotland.

The Scottish programme was established with a total of seven fixed screening centres of which two are in Glasgow and one each in Aberdeen, Dundee, Edinburgh, Inverness and Irvine. Given Scotland's geography and population distribution, there was also a need for mobile units to take the screening service to women living at a distance from the main centres. Over the first few years of the programme, nine such mobile units were commissioned. There are currently 12 of these on the road and the fleet is gradually being replaced and refurbished.

Throughout the United Kingdom, the programme was supported by a very comprehensive system of audit and quality assurance as mammography is a slightly less than ideal screening test and requires very close supervision of performance at all stages to yield the results desired. In comparative terms, the Scottish screening programme has performed very creditably in regular comparisons with programmes elsewhere in the UK.

The South East Scotland division of the Scottish breast screening programme commenced operation on 1st June 1998 at which time the radiologists involved were Alastair Kirkpatrick, B B (Nicé) Muir and James Walsh. At that time all of them had other hospital commitments. The consultant radiologist staff was increased by the appointment of Melanie Chapman in 1997.

Jean Murray, a staff grade physician, also trained as a radiologist and takes part in film reading.

Radiotherapy and Oncology

Until the 1920s almost the only available treatment for cancer was surgery. From around 1925 onward, x-rays and radium became available, either for use on their own or as an adjuvant to surgery. Until the appointment of Robert McWhirter and the inception of the National Health Service, there was no separation of diagnostic radiology and radiotherapy. However, there are some ways in which the management of cancer differed.

Once an up to date radiology (including radiotherapy) department had been established in 1926, the board of management of Edinburgh Royal Infirmary turned its attention to the use of radium. Because of the difficulty in handling radium and its cost (a donation of £5,000 purchased half a gram of radium in 1929) the board considered the possibility of allocating a number of beds specifically for patients who required radium treatment. An opportunity presented itself in 1926 when Lady Mary Anderson, widow of a former treasurer of the Bank of Scotland, bequeathed her mansionhouse "Beechmount" on Corstorphine Hill to the Infirmary. After adaptation and enlargement at a cost of £11,000, Beechmount was opened to patients in October 1932 with 36 beds, as a radium annexe to the Infirmary.

In 1929 a Radium Trust and National Radium Commission were established in London, the Trust to hold supplies of radium and the Commission to deal with its distribution and use. The Royal Infirmary was selected as the centre in South East Scotland where radium therapy could be combined with teaching and research. In March 1930 the managers entered into an agreement under which the Commission, on the recommendation of Edinburgh University Faculty of Medicine, was to provide the Infirmary with a supply of radium, subject to certain conditions of use. Among these conditions was a stipulation that a scheme be drawn up jointly by the Infirmary and the University. Full records of treatment and follow-up were to be maintained and the Infirmary was required to accept and to treat properly accredited patients from any source. The selection of patients

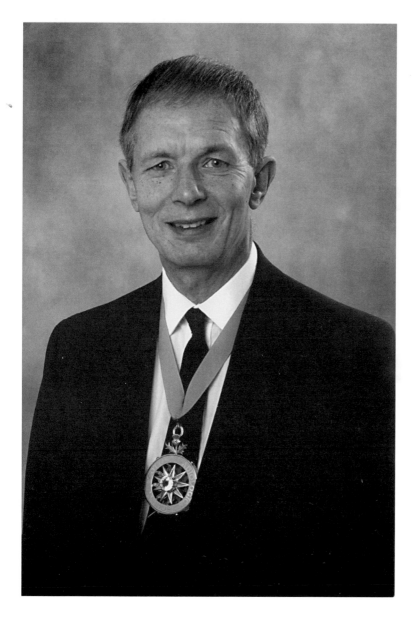

The Author. John F Calder (President of the Scottish
Radiological Society 1997–1999).

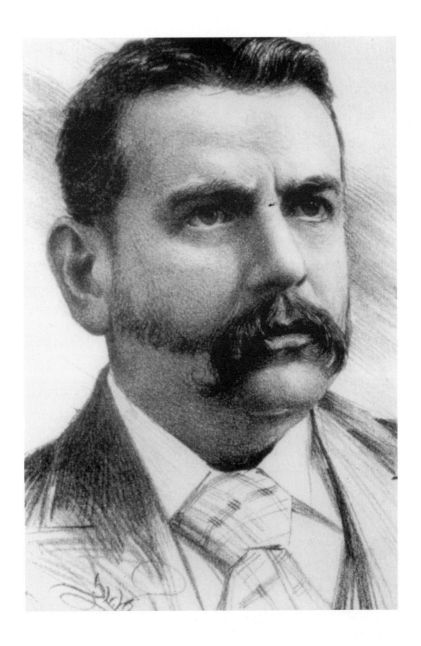

2. John Macintyre. Glasgow Royal Infirmary, 1895–1926.

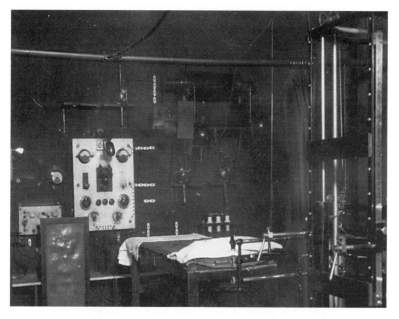

3. X-ray room. Glasgow Royal Infirmary, 1896.

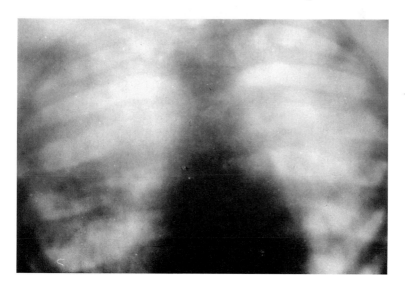

4. Macintyre's first x-ray of pulmonary tuberculosis.

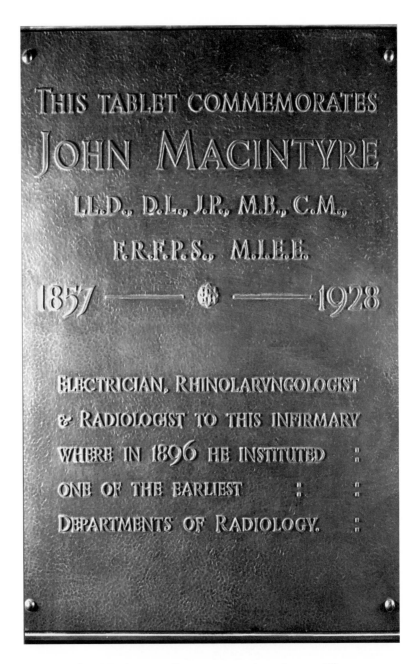

5. John Macintyre. Commemorative plaque. Glasgow
Royal Infirmary.

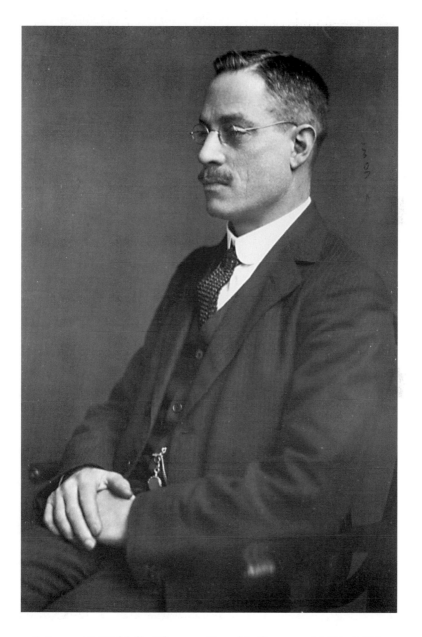

6. James R Riddell. Glasgow Royal Infirmary, 1902–1920;
Western Infirmary, 1920–1932.

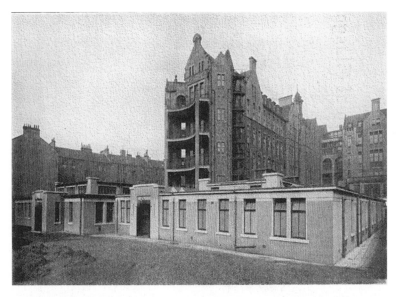

7. The new x-ray department, Western Infirmary, Glasgow
1930.

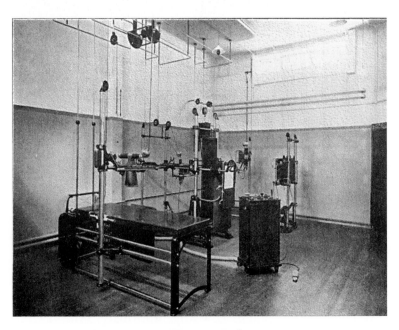

8. X-ray room Western Infirmary 1930.

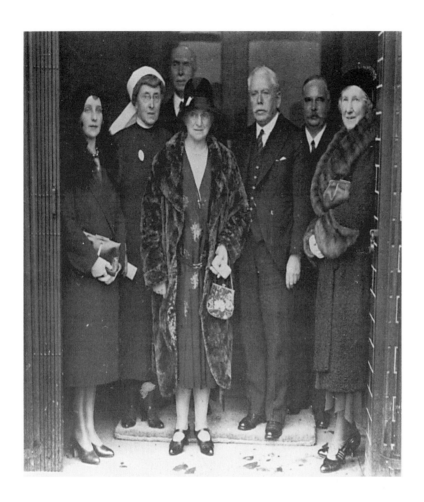

9. Opening of the new x-ray department, Western Infirmary, 1930.

Sir John Roxburgh   Sir Brian Kelly   Col Mackintosh
Miss Smith
Mrs McCredie   Mrs R D McGregor   Lady Nairn

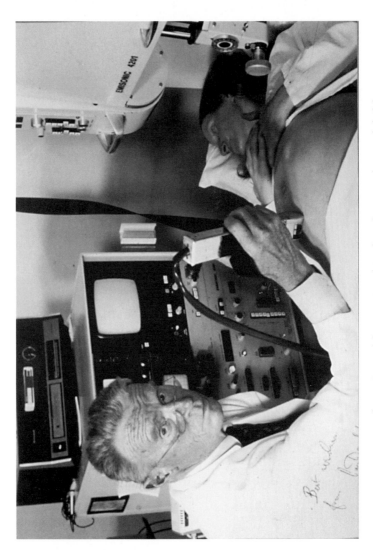

10. Prof Ian Donald scanning his daughter and grandchild.

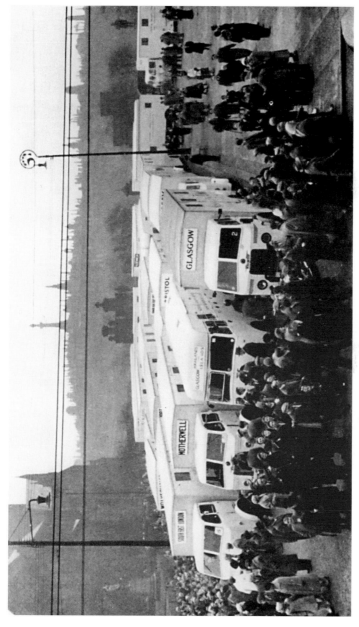

11. Glasgow Campaign Against Tuberculosis.

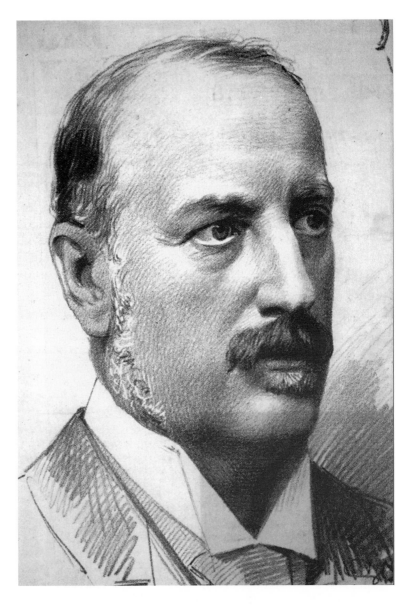

12. Sir George Beatson. Cancer Surgeon, Glasgow.

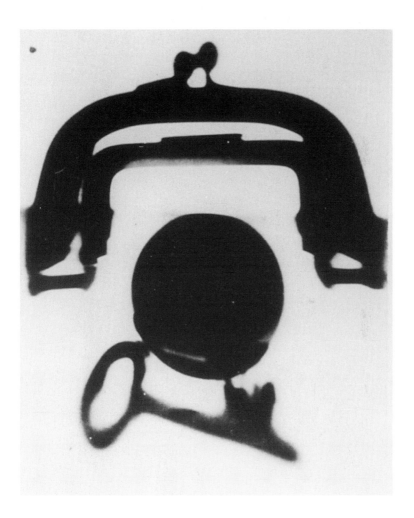

13. Dawson Turner's radiograph of a purse containing a
florin and key, 1896.

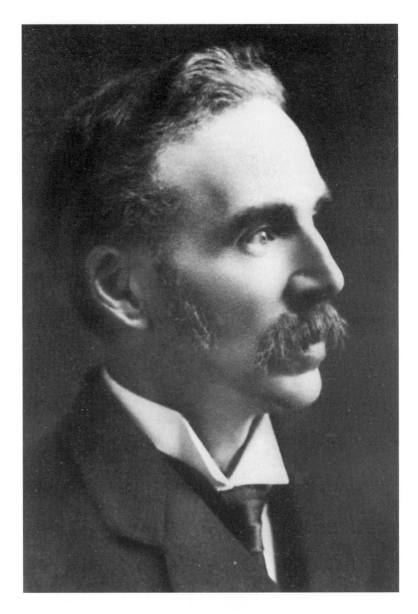

14. Dawson Turner 1898–1925

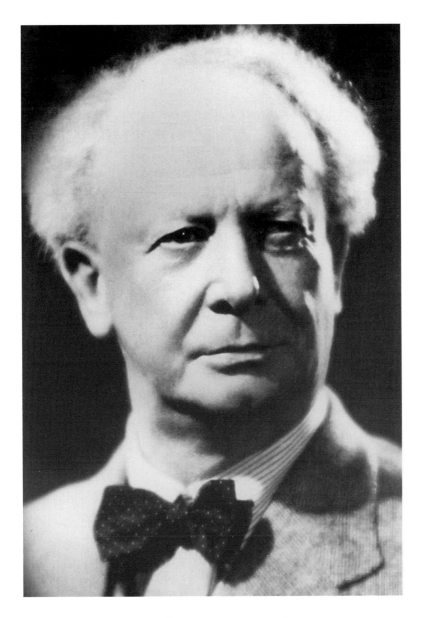

15. J Woodburn Morison 1926–1930

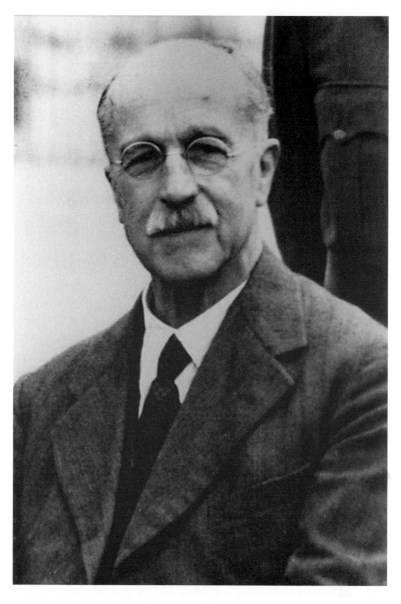

16. A E Barclay 1936

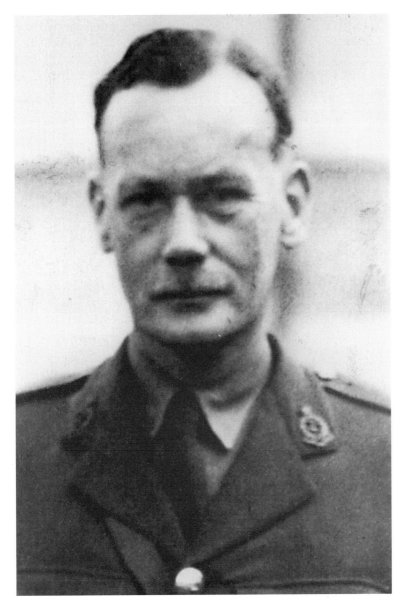

17. Duncan White 1930–1937

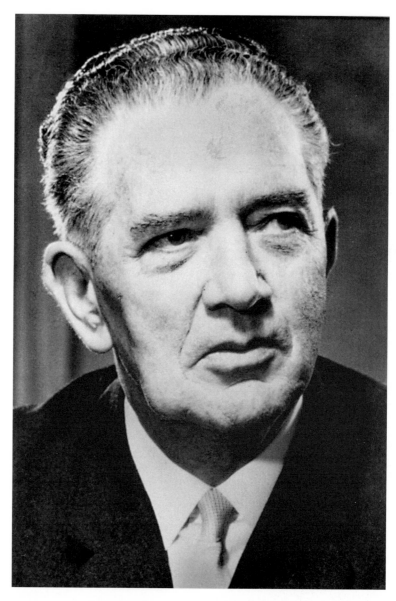

18. Robert McWhirter 1937–1945

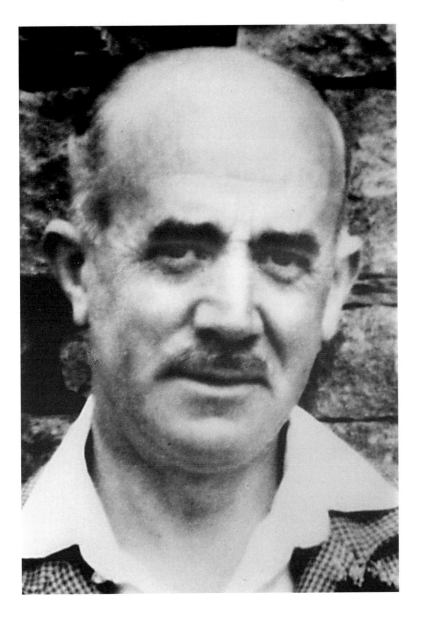

19. W S Shearer 1946–1957

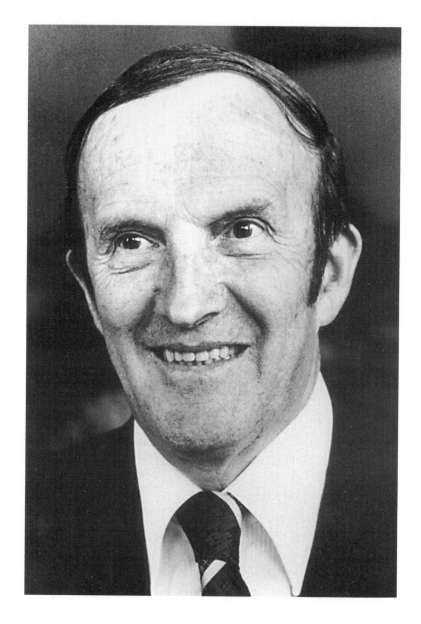

20. Eric Samuel 1958–1978

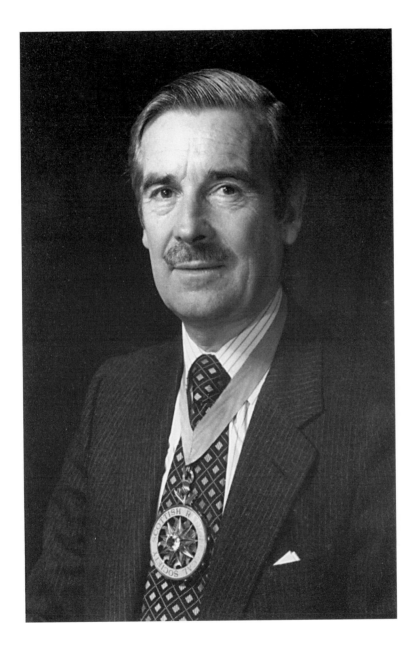

21. Tom Philp 1978–1986

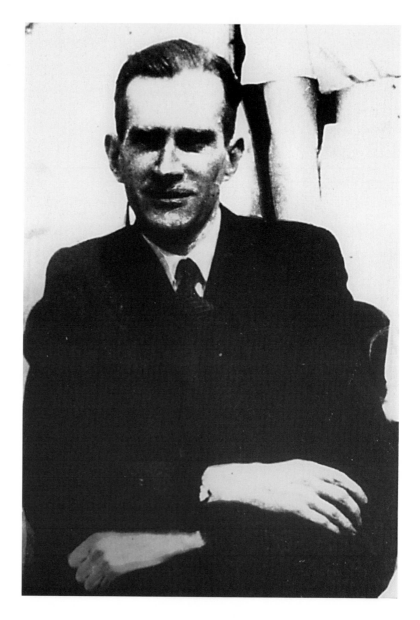

22. John Paton McGibbon. Royal Infirmary of Edinburgh,
1942–1952.

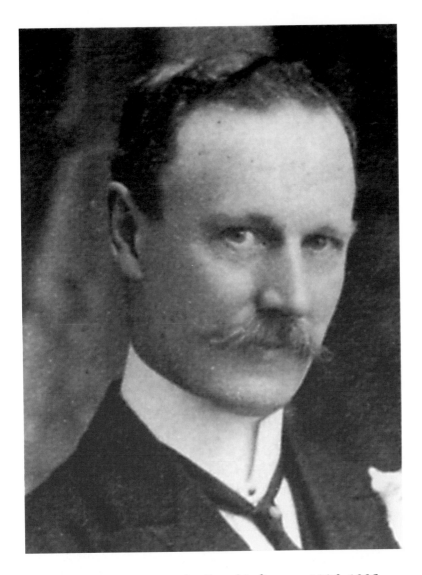

23. George Pirie. Dundee Royal Infirmary, 1896–1925.

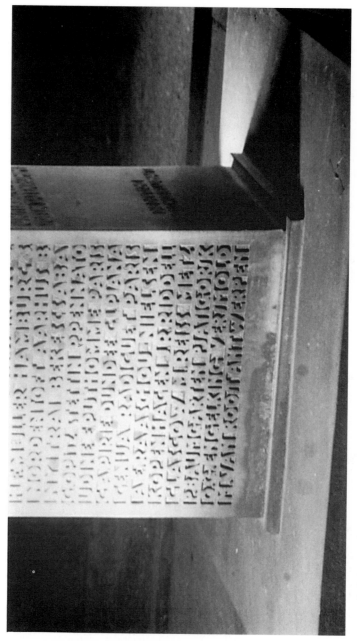

24. Martyrs' memorial, Hamburg showing the names of James R Riddell and George Pirie.

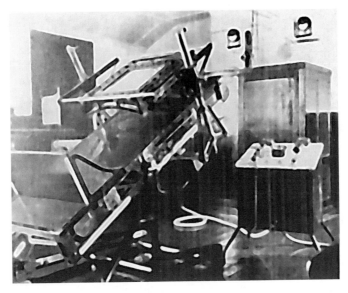

25. X-ray room, Lochmaben Sanatorium, 1927. The room
had previously been the kitchen.

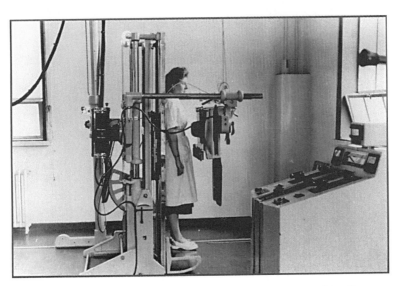

26. X-ray room, Queen Margaret Hospital, Dunfermline,
1949.

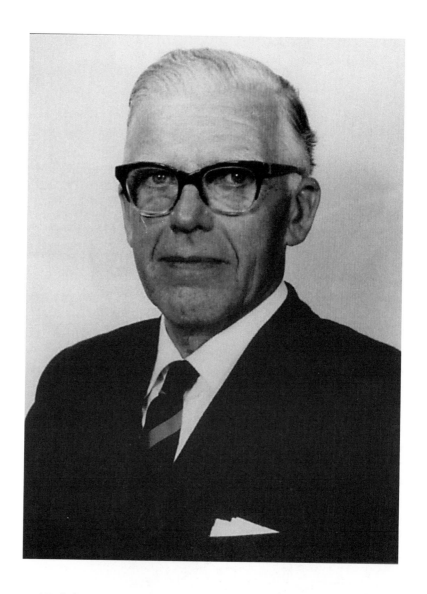

27. John Innes. Victoria Infirmary, Glasgow 1946–1972.

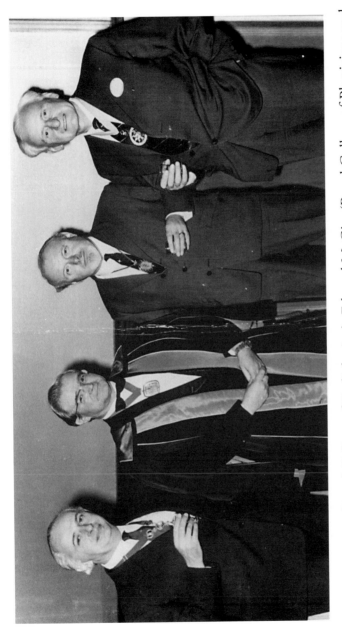

28. Robert Steiner (Royal College of Radiologists), Edward McGirr (Royal College of Physicians and Surgeons of Glasgow), Howard Middlemiss (Royal College of Radiologists) and Hunter Cummack (Scottish Radiological Society) at the establishment of the Standing Scottish Committee.

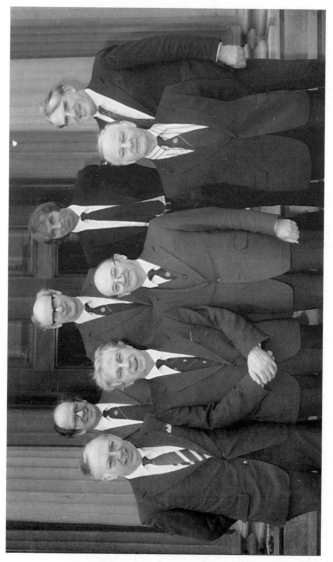

29. Some notable Scottish radiologists at a meeting in Glasgow, March 1985.
Tony Brewin   Bill Duncan   Mike Buist   Jake Davidson
Lewis Gillanders   TonyDonaldson   Bill Ross   Gerry Flatman

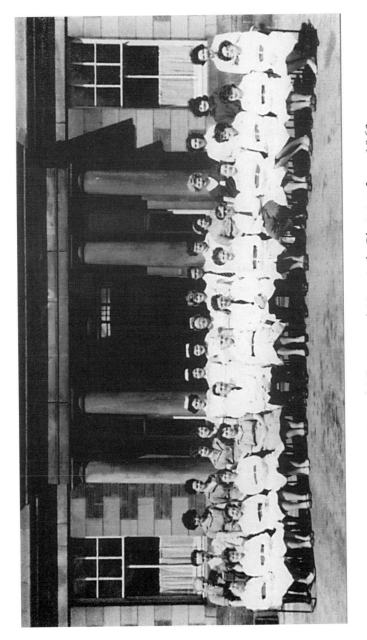

30. X-Ray staff Southern General Hospital, Glasgow, June 1963.
Wilson James, Jake Davidson and Kenneth Grossart are in the front row.

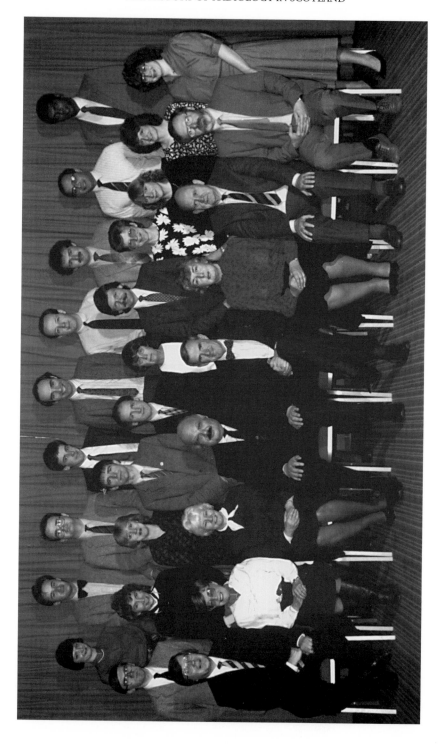

31. Western Infirmary, Glasgow x-ray staff at Ellis Barnett's retiral in January 1987.
Back row: Hilary Dobson Alan Ramsay John Roberts John Straiton Colin Campbell
 Richard Edwards Sutherland McKechnie R Mahraj J Namasivayam
Middle Row: Brian Mucci Fiona Howie Anne Hollman George Stenhouse
 Nigel McMillan Patricia Morley Michael Cowan Barbara Dall Susan Ingram
 Wilma Kincaid Grace Hare
Front Row: Ramsay Vallance J McDermid Dorothy Rigg Ellis Barnett Jake Davidson
 R McKinnon Albert Aylmer Fred Adams

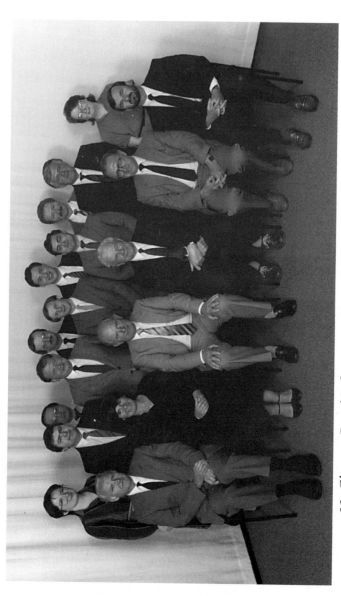

32. Glasgow Royal Infirmary staff at J G Duncan's retiral in 1987.
Back row: Fat Wui Poon Russell Pickard Allan Reid Patrick Walsh
Middle row: Fiona Gardner Julian Guse Alastair Forrester Grant Baxter Michael Dean Ian McLeod Jean Lauder
Front Row: Derek Lightbody Dorothy Anderson Nimmo McKellar James Duncan Brian Moule Ian Stewart

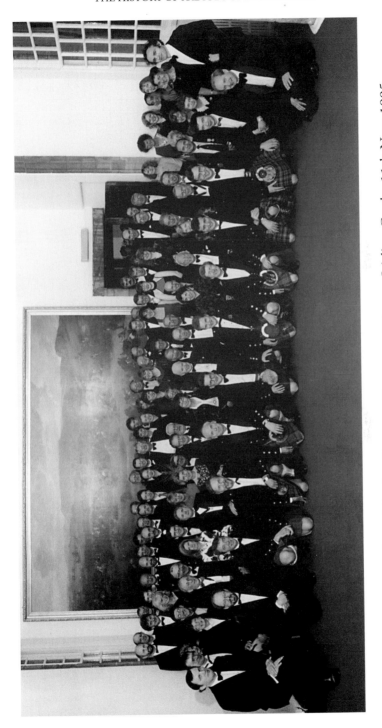

33. Scottish Radiological Society Röntgen Centenary Dinner, Stirling Castle, 11th Nov. 1995.

was left to the discretion of the hospital, guided by the principles of need and suitability of the patient for radium treatment.

When Beechmount first opened, many patients received treatment at the Infirmary then went to Beechmount for convalescence. This soon changed and most of the treatment was given at Beechmount though some who required deep x-ray therapy had to endure the discomfort of repeated ambulance journeys between the two centres. In 1934 history was made when Beechmount became the first hospital outside London to receive what was then known as a radium "bomb". The surgeon in charge at Beechmount was J J M Shaw. He was a greatly admired general surgeon who had a particular interest in the application of radium and x-rays to cancer treatment. His abilities as an administrator were instrumental in his appointment to the National Radium Trust and Commission. In 1934 he took a leading part in setting up the Cancer Control Organisation for Edinburgh and South East Scotland. His assistant was Margaret C Tod, an associate surgeon who made an outstanding contribution to the work at Beechmount before going on to be assistant and later deputy director of the Holt Radium Institute in Manchester. Beechmount continued to be used principally for treatment by radium until 1939 when on the outbreak of war, it became an auxiliary hospital and its radium was removed to the Infirmary for safe keeping.

As mentioned in the history of diagnostic radiology at the Royal Infirmary, A E Barclay had acquired Metropolitan-Vickers deep x-ray apparatus in 1935 and the department was further modernised and re-equipped by Robert McWhirter when he took over in 1936. Soon after his appointment to the Forbes Chair of Medical Radiology in the University of Edinburgh in 1946, McWhirter was instrumental in separating radiotherapy from diagnostic radiology. He persuaded the managers, in accordance with a National Radium Commission recommend-ation, to appoint a physicist to the department to undertake scientific calibration of the x-ray tubes and of the radium "bomb", advise on repairs to radium containers and test for leakages. This physicist was C A Murison who moved from the Royal Infirmary to the Western General Hospital in 1955.

From 1946 Robert McWhirter concentrated on radiotherapy. He had had many successes in treatment of cancer of the brain, thyroid and bone. It was, however, his management of breast cancer that established his reputation. He convinced his colleagues that radical mastectomy could be replaced by simple mastectomy and radiotherapy. He had more difficulty in convincing a largely hostile audience at the Royal Society of Medicine in London in 1948 but results from others soon confirmed his work. He was largely responsible for establishing the Radiotherapy Institute (later the department of clinical oncology) at the Western General Hospital in 1954. He was a gifted and stimulating teacher who attracted many postgraduate students to his department. Many of them subsequently became heads of department in Britain and throughout the world. Dr McWhirter played a leading role in the Faculty of Radiologists, culminating in his presidency in 1966. He was also elected a Fellow of the Royal Society of Edinburgh and was awarded the Gold Medal of the Society for cancer relief in 1985. In 1963 he received the CBE for his services to radiology and clinical oncology. Robert McWhirter died of a stroke in his own hospital in 1994 just before his 90th birthday.

A significant appointment in 1947 was that of William M Court Brown. His work on the hazards of radiotherapy contributed to the Medical Research Council's establishing the Clinical Population and Cytogenetics Unit. He had the foresight to appreciate the significance of the ability to describe the human genome in 1956 and employed three biologists to examine the effects of radiation on the genome. This eventually led to studies of the human karyotype in the population.

A feature of Edinburgh radiotherapy was the development of specialist interests in particular tumour sites. Of Prof McWhirter's colleagues, Mary Douglas specialised in gynaecological cancers, James Pearson developed treatment of oesophageal cancer, James McLelland treated brain tumours, Gordon Ritchie had a particular interest in lymphoma and John (Archie) Orr made major contributions to the later neutron trials with emphasis on head and neck cancers. Allan Langlands collaborated with the surgeons in the management of breast cancer.

In 1954, the year the department opened, around 2,300 patients were referred of whom approximately 1,300 were given radiotherapy. About 200 of these had benign conditions, mainly ankylosing spondilitis. The acquisition of megavoltage therapy in 1955 led to an increase in the number of cases of malignancy treated which rose from 1,000 to 1,500 within five years.

William Duncan succeeded Robert McWhirter as professor. In collaboration with Sidney Arnott, he instigated a series of meticulous trials on the effects of neutron therapy. Follow up revealed that neutron therapy was no better than photon irradiation and also caused considerable destruction of normal tissue. Professor Duncan was awarded the Röntgen prize by the British Institute of Radiology in 1987. He left Edinburgh when he was appointed head of the radiotherapy department in the Princess Margaret Hospital, Toronto. After five years he returned to Edinburgh and was re-appointed to the chair (William McKillop had been professor in the interim). Around this time he welcomed Prof John Smyth to the department of medical oncology and did everything to ensure that this venture was a success. Bill Duncan retired in 1995 and was replaced as professor by Allan Price.

Hugh McDougall came from Dundee in 1986, became head of department in 1990 and clinical director in 1994. In order to upgrade the patient care facilities, he obtained £1 million grant from the Cancer Relief McMillan Fund and further funding from Lothian Health Board.

The other consultants currently in post and their special interests include Grahame Howard in urological cancer, Valerie Cowie in gynaecological cancer, Anna Gregor in neurological, lung and paediatric cancers, Ian Kunkler in breast cancer, Catriona McLean (who has a job share with Felicity Little) in colo-rectal cancer, Hamish Phillips in upper gastro-intestinal cancer and Lillian Matheson in lymphoma.

With a further change in the management structure in 1999, Grahame Howard took over from Hugh McDougall and has the title of patient services director. The Edinburgh department has responsibility for oncology services to the Lothians, Fife, the Borders and Dumfries and Galloway.

4

Aberdeen and Grampian

Aberdeen Royal Infirmary had an electrical department before 1895, but it was James McKenzie Davidson, an ophthalmologist, who took the first interest in the medical application of x-rays. His contribution is discussed in Chapter 1. The first medical electrician who can be considered a radiologist was John Levack. He shared an interest in the development of x-rays with McKenzie Davidson and installed x-ray equipment in his house in Golden Square. He was appointed medical electrician to the Royal Infirmary in 1896 when an x-ray department was established. The early workload involved electrical treatments as well as the taking of skiagrams and the performance of procedures under fluoroscopy. Additional space, staff and equipment were soon required. An assistant electrician, Clifford T Bell, was appointed in 1905 and remained in post till 1918. Levack took an early interest in medical education and from his appointment in 1896, arranged for undergraduates to receive instruction in the department. This contribution was recognised by his appointment as lecturer in 1919. Levack retired in 1931 and was replaced by Middleton Conon. At that time the department, then situated in the old Royal Infirmary in Woolmanhill, was housed in a single room. A second room was added at the same time as ultra-violet treatment was moved from the x-ray department.

In 1933 David P Levack was appointed assistant radiologist and the move to the new site at Foresterhill was being planned. In 1935 John Blewett, an Australian, was appointed head of department. David Levack continued as his assistant. In the same year, Harry Griffith was appointed physicist. Griffith and Blewett developed photographic monitoring of radiation workers. This was taken up nationally within a few years and is still in use today.

The move to Foresterhill finally took place in 1936. An outpatient department with facilities for plain film radiography remained at Woolmanhill. Almost as soon as it was built, the new department was too small to meet the increasing demand for diagnostic services and it was unable to expand further as it was surrounded on three sides by established departments. New equipment was installed for the then enormous sum of £10,000. In 1939 Dr Levack was called up for military service and Dr Blewett had to run the department single handed till John Innes arrived as his assistant. Dr Innes left in 1946 to become head of the radiology department at the Victoria Infirmary, Glasgow. He was replaced as assistant by Sandy Bain who later became a consultant in Inverness.

In 1948 the inception of the National Health Service coincided with the separation of diagnostic radiology and radiotherapy. This year also saw the beginning of radiology training in Aberdeen. A second year senior house officer was seconded from Edinburgh for 12 months. In the 1950s, contrast studies were still being performed with a simple fluoroscope. This gave difficulties in implementing new techniques such as angiography. These difficulties were further compounded by lack of space. In 1963 a new barium suite with image intensification, ciné-radiography and eventually closed circuit television solved the problem. The 1960s showed great advances in specialisation. These included angiocardiography, peripheral and selective angiography, originally by George Mavor then by Lewis Gillanders, paediatric radiology by Archibald Stewart and neuroradiology by Robert McKail, followed by A F (Sandy) MacDonald.

Lewis Gillanders was appointed in 1958 and eventually succeeded David Levack as head of department. He was one of Scotland's most influential radiologists and is perhaps best known for his introduction of the "Foresterhill" system for measuring workload, used throughout Scotland until recently. He was active in developing radiological training and was instrumental in starting the DMRD course in 1967. For his services to medical education, Lewis Gillanders was awarded a personal chair in 1997. He also played a leading role in the Royal College of Radiologists, becoming its representative on the General Medical Council and eventually Vice President. He retired in 1988 and was not replaced as professor till later.

Sandy MacDonald had trained in radiology in Edinburgh and, under the influence of Tony Donaldson, had taken a particular interest in neuroradiology. As well as practising neuroradiology, he started the clinical services in nuclear medicine, ultrasound and mammography. A man of strong convictions, he refused to become involved in the mammography screening programme when it was decided nationally that only one, and not two views should be taken. A change in policy in 1995 to take two views at the first visit has vindicated his stance. He became President of the Scottish Radiological Society in 1990. He retired in 1993 as he did not approve of NHS trusts which he saw as the first stage of a Thatcherite attempt to privatise the National Health Service. When he left, the main responsibility for neuroradiology was taken on by Olive Robb.

Ronald Mahaffy was appointed in 1964. He took a special interest in angiography which was later to lead to interventional angiography. He also introduced lymphography to the department.

In 1966 phase one of the new hospital at Foresterhill opened and the inpatient department moved there. Once again, not enough space was made available and the original department had to be retained for outpatients. An outpatient department still continued at Woolmanhill and radiography was carried out at the City Hospital. Michael Allan looked after these departments as well as acting as visiting radiologist to Banff, Orkney and Shetland. When he left in 1978 these duties were shared by the other radiologists who sometimes found their visits to Shetland prolonged by inclement weather. The opening of the department in 1966 allowed space for the development of an x-ray theatre for cardiac catheterisation and angiography and eventually for ultrasound and CT. The first CT head scanner was installed in 1976. Initial attempts to obtain a body scanner were thwarted on financial grounds. However in 1981 the Aberdeen Evening Express "Laser Line" raised a public appeal for the purchase of a gynaecological laser. When the appeal exceeded its target, it was continued until £300,000 was raised to purchase an Elscint CT scanner. Ironically, donations came from all over North East Scotland, including Inverness, which eventually had to raise another appeal to purchase its own scanner.

Ultrasound had begun in the obstetric department in 1967 and the original machine was transferred to the x-ray department.

Its rapid growth as an imaging technique led to the appointment of two new consultants in 1975. A P (Tony) Bayliss, who had been trained by Ellis Barnett and Patricia Morley in Glasgow, took over responsibility for general ultrasound and has greatly advanced its use, including interventional techniques. Jamie Weir, who came from London, had spent a six month fellowship in Sweden learning echocardiography and is one of the few radiologists to have this interest. He was also instrumental in the installation, planning and running of the CT scanning service in which he was joined later by Elizabeth Robertson. Jamie Weir has also been very active in the Royal College of Radiologists and in 1999 demitted office as Dean of the Faculty of Radiology and Vice President of the Royal College. He is currently Chairman of the Standing Scottish Committee of the College. He is co-author of an "Imaging Atlas of Human Anatomy" published by Mosby-Wolfe in 1997.

Perhaps the most significant development in Aberdeen is that of magnetic resonance imaging. In 1974 Prof John Mallard of the department of biomedical physics and bioengineering at the University of Aberdeen formed a team to build a nuclear magnetic resonance imager. This team, led by James Hutchison, produced a functioning scanner by 1980. It was the world's first body MRI scanner. (At the same time the University of Nottingham had developed a head scanner.) The first clinical service was developed by Francis W Smith who had also taken on nuclear medicine. Commercial production was begun by M&D Technology in Aberdeen but only a few scanners were made. As with other developments, such as ultrasound, Scotland has now lost the lead. Aberdeen Royal Infirmary's current MRI scanner, like those elsewhere in the country, has been supplied by one of the major x-ray manufacturers.

There have been significant developments in other fields, particularly interventional radiology. This was mainly developed by Jefferey K Hussey from the vascular service provided by Ronald Mahaffy. It now extends beyond vascular intervention into other areas, including biliary and colonic stenting.

When Lewis Gillanders retired in 1988 the post of professor was not filled immediately. An earlier attempt to form an academic department foundered when John Calder, appointed senior lecturer in 1980, resigned to return to Glasgow in 1986.

This was a time of economic stringency in the university and the post was not filled. However, in the late 1980s, Roland and Lilian Sutton agreed to sponsor an Academic Chair of Radiology in the University of Aberdeen. They supplied considerable funding for this and, consequent on their donation, "The Roland Sutton Academic Radiology Trust" was founded in 1989 with a remit to improve education and research in clinical radiology for the benefit of patients in the North East of Scotland. An initial attempt was made to fill the chair in 1990 and 1991 but the university did not appoint at that time for several reasons. At that point the university, under the auspices of its then Vice Chancellor, Professor George McNicol, offered a personal chair to Jamie Weir and he accepted. The Roland Sutton Trust is independent, is formed of members of the Grampian Health Board and the University of Aberdeen in equal numbers, has independent finance and accountancy and is chaired by Jamie Weir. It has supported academic radiology in Aberdeen over the last decade by providing secretarial, administrative, technical and medical support for the department of clinical radiology as a whole but is particularly associated with education, training and research. The trust continued to support academic radiology throughout the early 90s and was eventually successful in 1995 by the substantive appointment of Fiona Gilbert to a full academic chair. Her chair is entirely supported by the Roland Sutton Academic Trust in terms of salary. The academic department has been strengthened further by the appointment of two senior lecturers, Alison Murray and Fintan Wallis, and a lecturer, Ian Smith. In 1999 the University of Aberdeen appointed Gillian Needham Dean of Postgraduate Medicine with the result that three Aberdeen radiologists are now professors.

In addition to Aberdeen Royal Infirmary, radiological services are provided elsewhere in the city. The Royal Aberdeen Children's Hospital and the Maternity Hospital are on the Foresterhill site. The first specialist paediatric radiologist was Archibald Stewart. He was replaced by Elizabeth Stockdale who remains in post. Other Aberdeen Royal Infirmary radiologists provide a sessional commitment.

In the 1950s, neurosurgery and thoracic surgery were provided at Woodend Hospital. The radiological support was provided by

Robert McKail. Later, Woodend was the home of gastroen-terological, orthopaedic and geriatric services. Peter Ward and Jeff Hussey had sessions there. The re-organisation of the National Health Service in 1993 led to the formation of a new trust which separated Woodend administratively from the Royal Infirmary. Frank Smith was induced to go to Woodend by the provision of a new low field MRI scanner for orthopaedic work and Angus Thomson was recruited from Dundee. 1999 has seen another re-organisation and Woodend has combined with the other hospitals in the region to form the Grampian University Hospitals NHS Trust.

Dr Gray's Hospital, Elgin

The earliest reference to provision of x-ray services in Elgin is in 1902 when a decision to purchase was deferred on the grounds of the cost of £35 8s. Following a donation of £10,000 by James Shepherd of Burntisland, an extension to the hospital was built and x-ray apparatus finally installed in 1908 at a cost of £154 17s 6d. Dr Alexander, a visiting physician, took charge of the x-ray and electrical appliances but by 1912 had devolved responsibility for the department to Sister Briggs. In 1915 new equipment was ordered at a cost of £79 5s. In 1916 Dr Alexander was mobilised for war service and responsibility for the department devolved to the matron, Miss Fraser. She eventually died of epithelioma of the jaw, possibly radiation induced. In 1922 a new screen was acquired, but by 1927 the equipment was considered obsolete and dangerous and new equipment was ordered to the value of £503 14s. This comprised a high tension transformer, a universal couch and screening stand, a fluorescent screen, a Metalix tube, a Potter Bucky Diaphragm, as well as wooden frames, tubing, cassettes and intensifying screens.

In 1932 it was agreed that Alexander Coutts Fowler of Aberdeen would act as an advisory radiologist. He died in 1933 and the services of an external specialist were dispensed with till 1936, when David Levack of Aberdeen was appointed. When Levack was called up for military service, John Blewett of Aberdeen agreed to visit Elgin once a month for the duration of the Second World War.

With the inauguration of the National Health Service in 1948 Elgin was included in the North Eastern Region and services considered at a regional level. David Levack advised a weekly visit to Dr Gray's and it was also suggested that an Aberdeen trainee should have duties in Elgin, a situation which a training committee would no longer approve. However these arrangements were not passed on financial grounds. In the 1950s the workload continued to increase but the facilities were too cramped to allow examinations to be done at speed and waiting lists grew. Radiography continued to be performed by a nursing sister and it was not until the 1960s that a radiographer was employed. By 1969 a new x-ray establishment had been opened and clinics were held twice weekly.

In 1973 pressure from local practitioners on the board led to the appointment of the first full-time radiologist, Alexander Simpson. In 1984 ultrasound was introduced and in 1990 Kenneth Brown who had trained in Glasgow, was appointed second consultant. In 1993 Alex Simpson retired on grounds of ill-health and was replaced in 1994 by John Addison, who had trained in Aberdeen. Approval for a third consultant post was obtained in 1996 but this has never been filled on a permanent basis. In 1997 following a public appeal for a CT scanner which started in 1993, a new eight room department was opened to include a spiral CT scanner, computed radiography with a total new equipment cost of £1.8 million and transfer of some "nearly new" equipment from the old department.

Radiotherapy and Oncology

The first request for radium for therapeutic use in Aberdeen was made by John Levack but it was deferred by the directors of the Royal Infirmary following doubts about its effectiveness.

Aberdeen received its first allocation of radium on 1922 for the treatment of cancer of the uterus. John Cruikshank who had come to Aberdeen from Dumfries to the Georgina MacRobert lectureship in malignant disease in the department of pathology, was charged in May 1922 with the custody and administrative control of radium. He was given the title of "radium officer" and reported to the "radium committee".

The role of the Radium Trust and the National Radium Commission has been described in the chapter on radiotherapy in Edinburgh.

In 1930 a strengthened joint committee was formed in Aberdeen and W G Evans was appointed MacRobert Lecturer in Malignant Disease at the University and Director of Radium Therapy and Research at the Royal Infirmary, a post which he held till 1939. Harry Griffith whose work on personnel monitoring has been discussed earlier, became Aberdeen's first medical physicist and played a vital part in the development of radiotherapy before, during and after the Second World War. Evans and Griffith devised a radium "bomb" which, although not the first of its type, represented a significant achievement. When Evans departed in 1939, James Philip was appointed surgeon in charge of radium therapy with the remit to work in close co-operation with the radiologist in charge of the x-ray department. These events were to lead to the separation of diagnostic and therapeutic radiology although, until the inception of the National Health Service, radium therapy remained in the hands of the radium officer while the therapeutic use of x-rays remained the responsibility of the radiologist. In 1936 the then new x-ray department contained a 100kV therapy machine for superficial treatment and a 250kV unit. In 1950 an additional 250kV machine was purchased.

During the Second World War, safety regulations meant that radium had to be capable of removal from patients and put in safe storage 50 feet underground, within 10 minutes of an air-raid warning. This was not possible at Foresterhill where treatment was centred. The radium stock was stored in a borehole in Rubislaw quarry and a small quantity was stored for special patients in a concrete protected safe in the hospital at Torphins. Radium salt was transferred from Marischal College to a quarry at Cove, where a small plant was set up to supply not only Aberdeen but also Edinburgh, Glasgow and Newcastle.

The National Radium Commission was wound up at the inception of the National Health service and Aberdeen developed its own policy in relation to cancer control. In 1949 James Philip became adviser to the Regional Hospital Board and in 1950 David Levack relinquished radiotherapy to Ernest Ridley who became consultant in charge. Ridley was eventually responsible for the complete physical separation of the two disciplines and a new purpose built department which was completed in 1963, contained the first cobalt unit.

The need for a unified cancer service became apparent in 1949 from a report published on the outcome of treatment of malignant disease at Aberdeen Royal Infirmary between 1930 and 1943. Until then there had been no co-ordination of the various disciplines involved in the management of cancer. As in the rest of the country, medicine and surgery were organised on a unit basis and the treatment depended on the views of the individual "chief". Until 1950 the use of radium and radiotherapy remained in charge of different disciplines. As a result of planning and consultation by the administrative and medical staff of the Aberdeen hospitals and the Faculty of Medicine, the malignant diseases unit came into being in 1950. It was responsible for all matters pertaining to the Health Board's cancer services. This unit formed the basis of the establishment of a department of oncology in the 1970s. In 1972 the Standing Cancer Committee in Scotland urged that other Scottish regions establish a cancer organisation similar to that which had been in evidence in Aberdeen for the previous 20 years.

The unit contained 30 beds and was staffed by two consultant surgeons, one consultant radiotherapist, one part-time radiotherapist and one part-time medical assistant. In 1976 Tarun Sarkar arrived to join Ian Kirby as the second radiotherapist. The increased workload required the addition of a second cobalt unit in 1975 and a simulator in 1976. The cobalt units have in turn been replaced by linear accelerators.

In 1978 Andrew Hutcheon was appointed consultant oncologist to develop the non-surgical care of solid tumours and to augment the efforts of those working with haematological malignancies. Originally split between Woodend and Aberdeen Royal Infirmary, medical oncology is now concentrated in the Infirmary's site at Foresterhill as an amalgamated ANCHOR unit (Aberdeen and North East Centre for Haematology, Oncology and Radiotherapy). Staff numbers have increased to include a professor of medical oncology, two medical oncologists, four clinical oncologists and a specialist registrar.

5

Dundee and Tayside

Dundee Royal Infirmary

George Pirie, the founding father of radiology in Dundee, was joined in 1913 by George Milln, who came from the Royal Navy at Haslar. Milln was called up for service in the First World War and on his return went into independent practice. He died in May 1945. Dr Grant is recorded as having come to Dundee between the wars. He was killed in 1947 or 48.

T S Sprunt came from Edinburgh early in the Second World War and like other radiologists provided both a diagnostic and a therapeutic service. He was joined by Dr Fleming who remained only a short time in Dundee before returning to London. In 1946 Cameron Swanson was appointed. He developed radiotherapy at Dundee Royal Infirmary and was given beds at the nursing home in Elliot Road. He gave many years of distinguished service to radiotherapy and is still enjoying an active retirement. James Riley was appointed in 1948. He graduated from the University of Edinburgh in 1935, gained his FRCS in 1938 and was surgeon at Bridge of Earn Hospital for a brief period. Following wartime military service in the Far East, he developed skin lesions which prevented his return to surgery. After the war, he obtained the diploma in radiotherapy from Edinburgh. He devoted most of his professional life to work on the mast cell and became an international authority on this. He discovered that the mast cell is a storage site for histamine and showed that in allergic reactions, histamine is released from the mast cells. J Stewart Scott came from Glasgow to succeed Cameron Swanson as head of department. He was later succeeded as consultant by Phyllis Windsor. Sachi Das was appointed in the late 1970s. Hugh McDougall was appointed in 1982. When he left for Edinburgh in 1986 he was replaced by John Dewar, the current clinical director. Alastair Munro is professor of radiation oncology.

Cecil Pickard was appointed consultant in 1952 and was responsible for developing the diagnostic service, while Cameron Swanson concentrated on radiotherapy. Under Dr Pickard's guidance, a new department was designed which in its time was unique in its use of a "race track" layout. The new department with six rooms was opened by the Queen on 28th June 1955. The first cardiac catheterisation in Dundee was carried out in 1952 by K G Lowe of the department of medicine. When the new department opened in 1955 the first bi-plane ciné angiography in Britain was carried out using equipment built by Cecil Pickard.

George Howie was appointed consultant in 1960 and became actively involved with Derrick Dewar in angiocardiography in the investigation of congenital heart disease preparatory to surgery. He succeeded Cecil Pickard as head of department. Dr Dewar, who was also radiologist at Maryfield Hospital left for Dumfries in 1972. Dr Pickard was so dedicated to his work to the point that he developed a reputation for being "difficult". To some extent this reputation was inherited by his successor, Dr Howie. Frank Fletcher was appointed senior lecturer in 1964 and was later joined by John Soutar and Danny Sinclair, who brought experience in ultrasound and paediatric radiology from Edinburgh. First Dr Soutar then Dr Sinclair were to become heads of department in succession to George Howie.

In February 1997 the new teaching hospital and medical school at Ninewells were opened by the Queen Mother. Although most of the department moved to Ninewells, Dundee Royal Infirmary remained open till 1998 with neurosurgery in particular remaining there. The radiology support for this department was mainly provided by Winton McNab, who was to become President of the Scottish Radiological Society in 1993. An EMI 1010 head scanner was installed at the Royal Infirmary in 1976 and the first scans were done in June of that year. By 1984 there had been major improvements in CT equipment and in its clinical application. To meet the demands for this in Ninewells, a public appeal from 1984 to 1986 raised £1.25 million and the first whole body scanner was opened on 1st October 1986. In

May 1987 the original EMI 1010 scanner at the Royal Infirmary was replaced by a Philips Tomoscan unit.

Other developments in Dundee include angiography and interventional radiology, largely developed by William Shaw, who also became clinical director, and nuclear medicine, by Malcolm Nimmo, who was trained by Malcolm Merrick in Edinburgh. The first MRI scanner in Dundee, a Siemens 1 Tesla unit, was commissioned in December 1992. A second scanner has since been installed but funding has not always been available to staff it adequately. Graham Houston has been mainly responsible for cross sectional imaging and has organised a successful Scottish course in recent years. The MRI team has been further strengthened by the appointment of Declan Sheppard, a former Glasgow trainee, who returned to Scotland after two years in the United States where he gained MRI experience in the M D Anderson Cancer Centre and in the North Western Hospital, Chicago. The current clinical director is Alan Cook, who also runs the mammography service.

Perth and Angus

The radiology department at Perth Royal Infirmary was opened in 1945 and Alexander (Tubby) Robertson was appointed the first radiologist. He was also the medical superintendent and was in charge of physiotherapy. John McLeod was appointed consultant radiologist to Stracathro Hospital in 1944 and following National Service, was appointed to Bridge of Earn Hospital in 1950 and Perth Royal Infirmary in 1963. David Ritchie was appointed SHMO in radiology in 1958 and consultant in 1963. In 1963 John Miekle was appointed to Perth and Bridge of Earn. Following the retirement of Drs McLeod and Ritchie, Richard Murray and Peter Gamble were appointed consultants. Since John Miekle's retiral, and with the ever increasing workload and new developments, there have been several new consultant appointments. These consultants are Janet Flinn, Kenneth Fowler, Suzanne McClelland and Robert Pearson.

Stracathro Hospital near Brechin was expanded as an emergency medical service hospital in 1940. Adam Elektrovich, who had previously been professor at Krakow University, Poland and had been a protegé of Madame Curie, was the first radiologist.

He had already lost two fingers from exposure to radiation. When he retired in 1956 he was replaced by Dr White who died in 1957. He in turn was succeeded by Robert J C Campbell who retired in 1968. The appointment of Donald Sutherland in 1964 linked Stracathro Hospital with Arbroath. William Gibson was appointed in 1968, became President of the Scottish Radiological Society in 1991 and retired in 1999. John Tainsh was appointed in 1986.

6

The Rest of Scotland

The Rest of Scotland

Although most of the developments have taken place in the major cities, there has been radiological activity, some of it innovative, in many parts of the country since the late nineteenth and early twentieth centuries. This has accelerated in recent years with the opening of several new district general hospitals, often better funded than their city counterparts.

Inverness and Highland

The first x-ray machine in Inverness was purchased by public donation in 1907 for £432. It was installed in the newly created department of electricity and massage at the Royal Northern Infirmary. It was initially used for diagnostic purposes only but 1908 saw the start of its use for radiotherapy. In that year 82 patients were treated, mostly for inflammatory conditions and rodent ulcers. By 1913 this number had risen to 413. In 1920 a stock of radium was bought through a donation of £275, in 1925 an ultra-violet light source was installed and in 1930 electricity and massage were separated.

Before 1938 x-rays were probably taken by nurses and were read by Dr McFadyean, a local general practitioner. In Culduthel Isolation Hospital they were taken by Edward Johnstone, Medical Officer of Health, a thoracic physician and by the resident medical officer. It is also known that J Campbell Tainsh was a radiologist in the 1930s. In 1942 Raigmore EMS hospital opened. Dr Gottlieb from Poland became resident radiologist. He also served the Royal Northern Hospital both as diagnostic radiologist and radiotherapist. In 1947 he started an "X-Ray Therapy Register" which listed the names of patients receiving radiotherapy, their diagnosis and referring consultant.

In 1947 just before the start of the National Health Service, the Highland region with a population of approximately 200,000, had minimal radiological cover. Only in the Royal Northern Infirmary and Raigmore was there a full service. The radiologists at that time were J C Wood and Alexander Bain. Kenneth Mackenzie, a radiotherapist from Edinburgh, visited every two months. In 1950 James Sangster was appointed to Raigmore while Sandy Bain concentrated on the Royal Northern. In 1955 Hamish Innes was appointed, originally as senior registrar then subsequently consultant. By 1960 M W M (Monty) Hadley had been appointed and by this time, the Inverness radiologists covered the entire Highland region, carrying out visits to Stornoway, Skye, Thurso, Wick, Golspie, Dingwall, Nairn and Fort William.

In 1962 Kenneth Mackenzie, formerly visiting radiotherapist, left his post in Edinburgh and was appointed consultant. In 1970 he succeeded in persuading the Highland Health Board to build a radiotherapy department in the new outpatient building of Raigmore Hospital. A second hand cobalt machine was purchased and a new orthovoltage machine installed. Dr Mackenzie retired in 1977 and was succeeded by George Jardine. He subsequently retired in 1982 and in 1983 was replaced by Mumtaz H Elia. In 1988 major development took place with extension of the department and replacement of the cobalt unit by a linear accelerator. A radiotherapy planning computer and a therapy simulator were installed for the first time. David Whillis was appointed consultant in 1991. A dedicated in-patient oncology/ haematology unit was opened in 1997.

From 1970 onwards, there were major developments including the installation of image intensification in central and some peripheral hospitals and the introduction of arteriography, venography, lymphography, mammography and interventional radiology. Teleradiology and ultrasound commenced with the help (in peripheral hospitals) of radiographers trained in their use. By 1978 Frank Williams had joined as consultant radiologist. The introduction of medical physics allowed the development of nuclear medicine. Most of the services were becoming concentrated in the new hospital at Raigmore. Monty Hadley became President of the Scottish Radiological Society from 1981 to 1982. He retired when the Royal Northern closed and was replaced by George Aitken. In the early 1980s a public appeal was started for the purchase of a CT scanner and eventually a sum of £1.25 million was raised.

David Nichols was appointed in 1986. A former Aberdeen trainee, he had spent some years in Vancouver from where he brought valuable interventional skills to Inverness. The consultant team has been enlarged to cope with the ever increasing workload and now includes David Goff, Peter Hendry, Alistair Todd and Andrew McLeod. They cover the entire Highland region except the Western Isles.

In 1990 Ian Riach was the first consultant radiologist appointed to the Western Isles. He was based originally at the Lewis Hospital till it was replaced by the new Western Isles Hospital in Stornoway in 1992. He took over the examinations, such as bariums and ultrasound formerly carried out on a visiting basis from Inverness and also reporting which had previously been performed by the consultant physician and surgeon on their own referrals. The appointment of a consultant radiologist has allowed an improvement in the level of service in the Western Isles. A spiral CT scanner was installed in 1998. Radiology is also provided at Daliburgh Hospital in South Uist, where there is a single roomed x-ray department and ultrasound. The radiologist visits monthly, mainly to perform ultrasound. The film reporting is now done daily via a teleradiology link with the Western Isles Hospital.

Fife

Dunfermline Cottage Hospital opened in 1894. The first x-ray apparatus was donated as early as 1898 when Mrs Louise Carnegie presented "a complete set of apparatus for the production of the Röntgen rays". For many years James Norval, a local photographer, was the custodian. He was followed by other operators, then radiographers. A visiting radiologist was not appointed till 1940. In 1909 a cable was laid to the hospital and new equipment provided by Robert Walker, President of the Managers, was activated by the "powerful electric current" supplied by the Fife Electric Power Co. This x-ray set, which cost

£135 8s improved exposure times, for example for a hand, from 15 minutes to 30 seconds. In 1930 x-ray equipment was donated to Dunfermline and West Fife Hospital by Mrs W B Street of Cowdenbeath in memory of her daughter Effie who had died aged 25. In 1949 there was further development of a new x-ray wing partly funded by a grant from the Carnegie Dunfermline Trust. In 1995 79,624 examinations were performed on 59,363 patients.

Whereas Dunfermline was the birthplace of Andrew Carnegie and benefited from funds supplied by the Carnegie Trust, Kirkcaldy was better known for the production of linoleum, one of the leading companies being owned by the Nairn family. In 1890 Mr Nairn gifted the new Kirkcaldy Hospital in gratitude to the townspeople who had contributed to the prosperity of his factories. In 1903 Michael B Nairn provided a powerful x-ray instrument for Kirkcaldy Cottage Hospital. The foundation stone of another hospital was laid in 1897, the year of Queen Victoria's diamond jubilee. Opened as Kirkcaldy Fever Hospital in 1899, this hospital was developed with a major tower block extension in 1967 and has become the present Victoria Hospital. In 1949 Peter Aitken was the first radiologist based in Fife. He became President of the Scottish Radiological Society from 1976 to 77. Andrew Dick was appointed consultant in 1966. He became consultant in administrative charge of diagnostic radiology services in Fife in 1986. He strengthened academic links by becoming lecturer in anatomy at St. Andrew's University.

Facilities in Kirkcaldy have been brought up to date with the recent acquisition of an MRI scanner.

Forth Valley

For many years, radiologists had joint appointments at both Stirling and Falkirk. The first radiologist who is mentioned as having worked at Stirling is G Jackson Wilson, who left for the Victoria Infirmary, Glasgow in 1929.

Following re-organisation in the early 1980s Stirling Royal Infirmary and Falkirk and District Royal Infirmary developed separately. There are modern departments with comprehensive facilities in both hospitals. Following further re-organisation in 1999, the departments have come together in a single trust.

Hazel Cunningham who returned to her native town in 1978 after three years as a consultant in Ayr is Stirling's longest serving radiologist. Peter McDermott in Stirling was the instigator of the Scottish clinical directors' group, which meets regularly to allow directors to exchange ideas and experiences. Dr McDermott represents this group on the Standing Scottish Committee of the Royal College of Radiologists.

Largely through the efforts of Jo Barry, Falkirk gained training recognition for radiology registrars. Mainly because of its central location, Falkirk and District Royal Infirmary hosts most of the meetings of the Scottish nuclear medicine group.

Lanarkshire

Hairmyres Hospital

The first x-ray machine, installed in 1923, was of the induction coil type. It was moved to another location in 1929 and a new couch and stand purchased to enable tele-stereoscopic films to be taken. By 1930 296 patients had been filmed. Lipiodil was being used as a contrast agent and in the same year, 19 barium enemas were carried out by clinical staff. There was a progressive increase in radiological activity in subsequent years. The number of chest x-rays rose from 756 in 1930 to 1,763 in 1938. This prompted Dr J Johnstone, the medical superintendent, to appeal for more space and equipment.

The opening of the new treatment block in 1939 saw the beginning of the radiological department on its present site on the upper floor. At this time the Council agreed to purchase a new x-ray unit, a Siemens Kodiaphos condenser discharge unit which was installed by German engineers. They had to be repatriated on the eve of war via Sweden through the good offices of the Red Cross. The first radiographer, Sister McNair, was appointed in 1938. The name of the first radiologist was uncertain but it was probably Dr McWhirter who is recorded as being in post between 1939 and 40. J Hurrel was probably his successor. He in turn resigned in 1944 to be replaced by Robert McKail. When Dr McKail left for Aberdeen in 1950 he was replaced in 1951 by William Monroe. In the interim Dr J Donald, a patient in Ward 8, did the non-tuberculous film reporting.

Dr Monroe stayed only a short time before returning to Kilmarnock. Dr Johnstone was still interested in the department and visited it at 4pm every week day to discuss administration with Sister McNair and to see the films of his own patients.

By 1952 the number of tuberculosis patients had fallen and the general workload increased. The need for further radiological cover was made even more necessary by the growth of the new town of East Kilbride. The chairman of the governing Western Regional Hospital Board, Sir Alexander McGregor, expressed the opinion that a better service could be provided in many peripheral hospitals by linking departments with those in teaching hospitals. As a result, J Z Walker of Glasgow Royal Infirmary was appointed part-time consultant in 1952. Dr Walker was only able to visit Hairmyres occasionally and a considerable amount of the work was carried out by registrars from Glasgow Royal. The main consultant input was provided by Sidney Haase who also had other commitments. Eventually in 1964 Murray Strathern became full-time consultant. He was a modernising influence and set about installing new equipment such as automatic processors, floating table tops, automatic exposure and AOT changers. The main x-ray department became equipped for angiography. Isobel Gray-Thomas joined the staff as assistant radiologist. Dr Strathern moved to Greenock in 1966 and Robin Freeland became radiologist in charge. Under his influence further improvements including image intensification, took place.

Following the break up of the Western Regional Hospital Board, Hairmyres came under the control of Lanarkshire Health Board. Robert Corbett was appointed consultant in 1976 and Rosemary Weir in 1977. Bobby Corbett was Honorary Secretary of the British Institute of Radiology from 1993 to 1996 and was elected President of the Scottish Radiological Society in 1999. Robin Freeland left in 1977 to take charge of the radiology department in the new Monklands Hospital. Isobel Gray-Thomas, by this time a consultant, retired in 1979 and was replaced by Marion Walker. She in turn left for Fife in 1985 and was replaced by Sam Millar. Fatma Mohsen was appointed in 1983, shortly after the CT scanner had been installed.

Coincident with the increase in staff was extensive modernisation of equipment. The first ultrasound machine was installed in 1977 and a new room built in the accident and emergency department. It was expanded more recently to house mammography and orthopantomography. The most significant development was the provision of a CT scanner, one of the first in Scotland and ahead of many city teaching hospitals. In 1980 Hosni Yosef, visiting radiotherapist, was approached by Mrs Ilse Youngman, a grateful patient, who wished to do something for the hospital. Together with John Douglas, consultant surgeon, they inspired the staff and public to raise funds for the scanner. By 1982 £1 million had been raised. On the day the contract was to be signed, snow had virtually put paid to all movement in England. Before a new date could be arranged, a new and significantly improved scanner was announced. Mrs Youngman insisted successfully that the new model be supplied at the original price. When the original scanner was replaced by a Toshiba helical scanner, Ilse Youngman was asked to perform the opening ceremony.

In 1992/93 the department performed 49,430 procedures. When the Hamilton/East Kilbride unit of the Lanarkshire Health Board formed in 1993 the x-ray departments of Hairmyres and Stonehouse Hospitals joined. William Campbell had been radiologist at Stonehouse since 1968 but died in the early 1980s. However since 1976 radiologists had had sessions in both hospitals. In addition to those already mentioned, the current radiologists are the present head of department Fiona Gardner, Clifford Murch and, part-time, Fiona Howie and Angela McCallum. Rachel Connor rejoined the department in March 2000 after a brief period at the Victoria Infirmary, Glasgow. Hairmyres Hospital is currently being re-built on site, funded by a private finance initiative. The new hospital is scheduled to open in 2001.

Law Hospital

The present Law Hospital has been developed from old war time pavilions, built near Carluke. Little is known about its radiological facilities before 1962. At that time William Dempster and Matthew Leach were the radiologists. Leach became ill and was given a sinecure post at Strathclyde Hospital. This left William Dempster and later William Mowatt, on a sessional basis, to cover the work. They were joined later by John Bell and these three were recorded as being in post in 1972. This was a time of expansion and acquisition of new equipment, much of it obtained through Dr Dempster's powers of persuasion with the Western Regional Hospital Board. Further changes were to occur in Lanarkshire with the opening of Monklands Hospital in 1977. Dr Mowatt gave up his sessions to go to Monklands and the same year, Edward J McKay and Dhirendra K Pattnaik were appointed. Both were later to retire in the mid 1990s on grounds of ill-health. Mohammed El-Sayed joined as consultant in 1986 and is still in post. Before they retired successively in the late 1980s and early 1990s William Dempster and John Bell had carried a large part of the ever increasing workload and were in turn head of department. John Roberts joined the department in 1998 and is the current clinical director. In addition to those mentioned previously, his colleagues are Marie Callaghan, Barbara Macpherson, Susan Reid, Desmond Alcorn and Mustaffa Fleet, all appointed since 1994. Law will soon be replaced by a new hospital on a greenfield site, financed like Hairmyres by PFI.

Monklands Hospital

When Monklands Hospital opened in 1977 Robin Freeland came from Hairmyres to take charge. He was joined at the same time by William Mowatt. Dr Freeland's health was poor and soon Dr Mowatt was in effective charge, eventually taking over when the former retired in 1982. James Johnstone became a consultant in 1978 but had to retire later on health grounds in 1999 and died later that year of colonic carcinoma. Ruth Holden, appointed in 1979, was the driving force behind Monklands' accreditation for registrar training, the first peripheral hospital in the west of Scotland to obtain such recognition, although Greenock had a registrar for a short time in the early 1970s. Kenneth Wallers succeeded as clinical director when William Mowatt retired in 1999. Other consultants currently in post are Kenneth Hughes, Julian Guse, Michael Gronski and Gordon Dewar.

Argyll and Clyde

Paisley

It has already been mentioned in the chapter on Glasgow that James Riddell, then of Glasgow Royal Infirmary, acted as consultant to the Royal Alexandra Infirmary at the beginning of the twentieth century and so there must have been an x-ray department at that time. It is known that Dr Stirling who retired in 1973 was a consultant radiologist at the Infirmary. Other consultants were A Stevenson who retired in 1977, J McLean who retired in 1984 and J McCavena who died the same year. When the new Royal Alexandra Hospital opened in 1987 J Gray Paterson moved there from the old infirmary. He retired in 1988. The Royal Alexandra Hospital has a spacious well equipped department and is a major improvement on the old infirmary. It has the only CT scanner for the region. The present consultants are Carole Alexander, Lester Cram, Mary Stevenson, Marie-Louise Davies, Joseph Negrette, Alan Wallace and Callum Adams.

Greenock

Greenock was among the first towns in Scotland to have x-ray apparatus. Mr Matthew Blackwood of Port Glasgow donated his own equipment in 1899. He was given the appointment of honorary x-ray demonstrator in recognition of his services and x-ray apparatus was purchased and installed to replace his original primitive machine. Radiological, and indeed all medical services in Greenock, Gourock and Port Glasgow were fragmented and distributed among several smallish hospitals including Greenock Royal Infirmary (surgery and A&E), Gateside and Larkfield Hospitals (medicine) until the opening of the new Inverclyde Royal Hospital in 1979 allowed centralisation of services and justified the provision of a fully developed x-ray department. In 1966 Murray Strathern came from Hairmyres as consultant radiologist and was joined by John Galloway in 1975. He subsequently left for Vale of Leven Hospital in 1988. Dr Strathern retired in 1993. The current radiologists are Patrick Walsh, Alan Ramsay, Peter Kelly and Robert Shaw.

Vale of Leven

Vale of Leven had the distinction of being the first new hospital to be built in Britain after the Second World War. Tom Cowie was the radiologist involved in the design of the x-ray department which opened in 1954. He had the complete co-operation of the design team in constructing a workable small department. From the beginning, general practitioners had direct access to x-ray facilities, quite an innovation at that time. Dr Cowie originally worked four sessions in addition to his commitment at Glasgow Western Infirmary. An extra session was added after two years and was generally covered by registrars from the Western. The complexity of the work increased to include angiography, using a simple cassette tunnel for serial films made by a local joiner, who also designed an extremely good chair for micturating cystograms.

By the end of the 1950s, the work had expanded to the extent that it could not be covered on a sessional basis. Tom Cowie gave up his sessions to concentrate on cardiovascular radiology at the Western Infirmary. Ben McKee was appointed full-time consultant radiologist in 1963. His contract included duties at Duntocher Hospital and clinics in Dumbarton and Oban. John Galloway came as a second consultant in 1988 and when Dr McKee retired, he was replaced by Irene Jackson, who had had a varied career before taking up radiology in 1980. She worked in Australia and Canada before returning to Scotland in 1969, spent several years in Blood Transfusion then took an interest in mammography under the influence of Wilson James at the Southern General Hospital. This encouraged her to become a radiologist and she took her fellowship in 1985 at the age of 50. After a comparatively short radiological career, she retired in 1995. John Galloway retired the same year and since then, has taken up a part-time post at Lorne and Islands Hospital, Oban, the first radiologist to be based there. After their retiral, a consultant post was filled for a short time by John Zachary. Iain McGlinchey, who was appointed in 1997, is currently the only radiologist, the other post having proved difficult to fill for more than temporary periods.

Ayrshire

Medical and radiological services in North Ayrshire were originally provided at Kilmarnock Infirmary. Dr McCrorie is thought to have been the first radiologist. He was succeeded by R M C Crawford who was a visiting radiologist from the Southern General Hospital in Glasgow.

In 1982, a new hospital opened at Crosshouse. The radiologists at that time were James Smith, Patrick Crumlish and Brian Stanton. Dr Crumlish succeeded Dr Smith as clinical director. He was in turn succeeded by Morag McMillan. Six consultant radiologists at Crosshouse, in a modern well equipped department which includes CT and MRI scanners, provide a comprehensive service for North Ayrshire.

Medicine and radiology in South Ayrshire were much more fragmented and were provided at Heathfield, Seafield Children's and Ayr County Hospital in Ayr and at the large wartime pavilioned hospital at Ballochmyle. The radiologists were Dr Mackie who retired in 1969, and Bertil Reid who died in 1971. Dr Mackie was succeeded by Michael Greenhill and Dr Reid by Douglas Russell.

In 1992 the new Ayr Hospital was opened by Prime Minister John Major. It provides a full range of services on a single site and was among the first hospitals in Scotland to install MRI. It is staffed by five consultants among whom Keith Osborne is notable as medal winner in both parts of the FRCR.

Dumfries and Galloway

The Royal Infirmary of Dumfries and Galloway at Nithbank acquired its first x-ray department in 1909. It was paid for by a donation of £122 4s by the parish of Mouswald near Dumfries. A physician, Dr Robson, became the first radiologist. In 1916 he expressed a wish to have gas supplied to the x-ray department for power not for lighting! In 1919 Dr Robson stated that he had treated free such patients as he thought were unable to pay. In 1921 the cost of x-ray plates was 10s 6d for a 10 x 12 inch plate, 7s 6d for an 8 x 10 and 5s for a half plate. An abstract from the treasurer's accounts for 1921/22 showed that £20 4s had been received from 45 patients for the use of x-ray apparatus. For comparison, 76 patients were seen in 1913, 61 in 1922/23 and 228 in 1923. In 1928 a new Coolidge tube was installed at a cost of £25.

At the inception of the National Health Service in 1948, Dumfries and Galloway had only one radiologist, John McWhirter, brother of Robert McWhirter of Edinburgh. There was one radiographer, Anne Webb who became superintendent in 1961. Most of the radiographers were recruited and trained locally until the Dumfries school of radiography closed in 1987. Dr McWhirter was consultant in administrative charge from 1947–1961. He was succeeded by Lockhart Frain-Bell who remained in charge for 25 years till he retired in 1986. Sam McCall Smith, whose father had been medical superintendent of the Victoria Infirmary, Glasgow, also joined the department in 1961 and stayed till he left for Peel Hospital, Galashiels in 1972.

The x-ray service in Dumfries and Galloway is conducted on an area basis and serves a population of around 150,000 in a region extending from Langholm to the Mull of Galloway. In addition to the Royal Infirmary x-ray departments were established in the Crichton Mental Hospital (now closed), which had a Banazetti tomogram for skull work in relation to pre-frontal leucotomies, Cresswell Maternity Hospital, Lochmaben sanatorium and cottage hospitals in Castle Douglas, Dalbeattie, Kirkcudbright, Newton Stewart and Stranraer. From 1961 a comprehensive service for general practitioners was established at these hospitals. Some GPs received training in elementary radiography and in the use of the cottage hospital equipment. The Garrick Hospital in Stranraer had its own radiologist, James Richard, a GP with the DMRD from before 1939 till he retired in 1973. After this his son-in-law, Robin Scott, a GP with some radiological training and experience acted as assistant radiologist with the support of consultants from Dumfries. By 1992 the number of x-ray examinations carried out at Stranraer had risen to 6833.

Lockhart Frain-Bell recounts some amusing anecdotes of what can happen in departments serving a largely rural area:

A ploughman from a farm in Galloway appeared at the department office the day after a barium meal asking for a bottle of the "stuff", the only medicine which had done him any good. He said he could not remember whether it came from a bottle of Bell's or Dewar's.

Another farm worker from Galloway sent the department a bill for some pounds for hay a week after a pyelogram. When he was at the x-ray department a cow had knocked down the byre door and eaten several bales of hay while the patient was delayed and had missed his bus because the examination had taken one hour.

Dr Frain-Bell was called urgently to Newton Stewart because the X-ray unit would not take films for an orthopaedic clinic. There was a smell of cooking in the room. When he removed the front panel from the control box he found that a mouse had eaten the insulation from the HT cable and it had shorted with the metal surround. The mouse was "cordon bleu"!

In the early 1960s a workman digging a trench outside the old Royal Infirmary noted a white porcelain box. He shouted to his mates "Ha, Roman remains" and, putting his pick through it, produced a blinding flash. The wooden handle saved him. The damage to the HT junction box put the department out of action for a day.

In Dumfries peripheral arteriography was started in the early 1970s using a Kodak industrial cassette in a home-made framework for changing films. It was placed on the floor with the patient on top, and the films were taken with an overcouch tube.

The new Royal Infirmary containing 424 beds and opened by the Queen in 1975 facilitated the development of an up to date radiology service which included ultrasound and mammography. The number of radiologists increased to four with the appointment of Derrick Dewar in 1972, David Jones in 1974 and George Watson in 1982. Dr Dewar retired in 1984 and David Hill was appointed in 1986. CT scanning was introduced in 1972. Penny Law was appointed in the same year because of the increased workload generated by the acquisition of the CT scanner.

7

The Scottish Radiological Society

On 10th October 1936 a meeting of the British Institute of Radiology was held in the Western Infirmary, Glasgow. Twenty two members were present. Eight meetings of this branch were held before the outbreak of the Second World War in 1939 and two further meetings were held in 1946 after the end of hostilities. The minutes of the pre-war meetings indicate a happy mixture of scientific discussion and social activities including golf where the venue was appropriate.

In 1946 in anticipation of the forthcoming National Health Service Insurance Act, it was agreed to ballot all the radiologists in Scotland on three proposals: Future meetings of radiologists resident in Scotland should be held 1. As a Scottish Branch of the Faculty of Radiologists proposed by Dr Robert McWhirter; 2. As a Scottish Branch of the British Institute of Radiology proposed by Dr Campbell Tainsh; 3. As a Scottish Radiological Society without affiliation to any other society proposed by Dr John Blewett. The first proposal was carried by a large majority. However, following an account of the attitude of the Faculty of Radiologists to a Scottish section and after considerable discussion, it was agreed unanimously that future meetings should be informal and unaffiliated to any other society.

The first meeting of an unaffiliated Scottish Radiological Society was held on 21st September 1946 with 15 members present. The chairman, Dr David P Levack of Aberdeen, an ex-POW, gave an account of mass radiography carried out by the German medical services in Oflag VIIIB in the spring of 1944. One thousand five hundred prisoners were examined. Only 10 cases of suspected pulmonary disease were found of which two proved to be open pulmonary tuberculosis. A description was given of the general difficulties encountered in getting the co-operation of the British camp authorities and the prisoners themselves and the unfortunate decision, against medical advice, to make the examination voluntary. Dr John Blewett read a paper on control of stray radiation using the photometric method. At the December meeting in 1946 Dr J B McWhirter of Dumfries pressed for action to be taken with regard to the supply of radium for the treatment of non-malignant gynaecological cases in local hospitals. He had been refused a supply by the Radium Commission on the grounds that there was lack of general x- ray control.

In 1947 with the National Health Service imminent, the members discussed again the advisability of affiliation to the Faculty of Radiologists or the British Institute of Radiology but decided to remain independent and to indicate to the Chief Medical Officer of the Department of Health for Scotland that the Society was constituted and prepared to enter into consultation with the department on matters affecting radiology and radiologists in Scotland.

An annual subscription of five shillings was agreed to meet all expenses.

The minutes of the next few meetings are succinct summaries of the scientific papers but in 1950 the question was raised as to whether the Society should have a politico-advisory role in addition to its scientific and social activities. Despite a dislike for medical politics expressed by some members, it was agreed to implement the original pre-war concept of a society which could represent the views of its members to the Scottish Home and Health Department. An executive council was set up with power to deal directly with matters political or of wide administrative interest to radiologists in Scotland. The first Chairman of the SRS Council was Dr J B King who, together with Prof R McWhirter, are revealed in the minutes as the guiding mentors of the Society in the early days of the National Health Service.

Two pounds presented to the Society in 1950, representing the balance of funds from the recent meeting of the International Radiological Society in Scotland, were directed towards general secretarial expenses in the SRS.

It is of interest to note that in 1951 the Society agreed to the principle of open access for general practitioners although over 20 years were to pass before this was fully implemented in the Health Service. In 1954 the constitution was amended to make

Council responsible to the Society. The first report of Council was circulated at the AGM in 1956.

Dinner at a private room in Gleneagles Hotel on 31st May 1958 after the AGM cost the members £1 2s 6d each. Those wishing to dance were charged a further half crown and were in addition required to wear formal evening dress!

A memorandum on the radiological services in Scotland prepared by the radiological services sub-committee in June 1958 showed that since the inception of the NHS, workload had increased by approximately 80% in a seven year period. Among scientific papers in 1960 was an early description of Crohn's disease affecting the large bowel, a talk by W Court Brown on chromosomal abnormalities in leukaemia with the suggestion that medical radiation played a part in the production of chromosomal abnormalities, and a description of ciné-radiography using the new image intensifiers — all original topics.

An annual lecture in memory of Dr John McGibbon, a greatly admired Edinburgh radiologist and a pioneer of cardiac radiology, was endowed in the early 60s. A grant from the European Association of Radiology following a successful meeting in Edinburgh in 1974 made it possible to re-endow the lecture in 1974 as a continuing academic memorial.

A presidential badge of office was presented in 1962 by a distinguished therapist, Dr J C Davidson of Glasgow, in memory of his mother. The design and manufacture of the insignia were specially commissioned by Dr Davidson from John Leckie Auld of Glasgow School of Art. A thistle suspension was introduced in place of a more medical symbol originally planned, to emphasise the Scottish identity. The centre consists of a perfect flawless crystal cut to scintillate light. This symbolised the sun, the principal source of light and radioactivity. Rays, both wave-like white and straight piercing gold, radiate into space bounded by a blue annullet of enamel. The original design placed the cabochon cut garnets on the front of the enamel but this was changed to the edge to accommodate the title of the Society. The garnets represent electrons in orbit as it was felt that this reflected some similarity in atomic structure and the solar arrangement of matter. A miniature replica of the badge is presented to retiring presidents of the Society.

In 1970 the Society acquired a permanent address at the Royal College of Physicians in Queen Street, Edinburgh with storage for its accumulating records and documents in the library of the college. The membership exceeded 200 in 1972 with approximately 150 diagnostic and 50 therapy members. In the early 1970s, impending re-organisation of the Health Service produced several important changes. In October 1970 the Scottish Committee for Medical Services (SCMS) resolved not to re-appoint the services sub-committees which had been in existence and had served a useful role since the early days of the NHS. Following publication of the Zuckerman report in 1971, which affected professional relationships between radiologists and radiographers, the question of a formal association between the Society and the Faculty of Radiologists (which was about to achieve collegiate status) was raised again as it appeared that advice on matters radiological in Scotland was likely to be sought from the Faculty. A Standing Scottish Committee of the Faculty was formed at the suggestion of Scottish radiologists to allow the Faculty to obtain a comprehensive opinion on relevant matters presented by the Department of Home and Health for Scotland and other bodies. This was of real importance because of the differences in the Health Acts in England and Wales and in Scotland. With the establishment of the Standing Scottish Committee of the Faculty of Radiologists, the early wish of the Society for association with the Faculty was eventually realised. The considerable achievement of Prof Howard Middlemiss and the Society's president, Dr J Hunter Cummack, in arranging a harmonious relationship, was timely. Shortly afterwards the Faculty achieved collegiate status and a royal charter. Dr Keith Halnan was appointed first Chairman of the Standing Scottish Committee which took over much of the medico-political business of the Society. One of the committee's first actions was to establish a radiographer liaison committee in Scotland. Methods of identifying workload in departments of radiology in Scotland were examined and the Foresterhill system adopted.

The role of the Society was reviewed again by its members in the 1970s in the light of its new association with the Royal College of Radiologists. It was agreed that the SRS had a special role in Scotland particularly through its scientific meetings. A Kodak prize was established in 1973 and awarded annually to the best paper given by a junior member at an annual meeting. The Bristol Myers prize was donated in 1987 for the best paper given by a junior radiotherapist. A Scottish Radiological Travelling Fellowship was funded by Nycomed in 1988 to support junior consultants and others wishing to undertake a period of study at a recognised centre of excellence. A later decision of Council broadened the scope of the fellowship so that any member is now entitled to apply.

Members and their families have enjoyed meeting in some of the most prestigious and beautiful locations in Scotland including Edinburgh Castle, Glasgow City Chambers, the ancient universities of Aberdeen and St. Andrew's and the Highlands. A Röntgen centenary meeting was held in Stirling in 1995, with the dinner in Stirling Castle attended by distinguished guests including the presidents of the Royal College of Radiologists, the British Institute of Radiology, the Scottish Royal Colleges and three Albanian radiologists who were visiting Glasgow at the time.

Joint meetings with radiologists in the North of England and in Ireland were arranged and the Society participated actively in joint meetings with the Royal College and British Institute of Radiology. A joint meeting with the University of Connecticut was held in Scotland in 1984. In recent years the Society has been more adventurous and overseas meetings have been organised in Cairo with the Egyptian Society of Radiology and Nuclear Medicine in 1992, in Cyprus with the Cyprus Radiological Society in 1994, and in Mombasa with the Kenya Association of Radiologists in 1997.

The Society now has its own web site with information about itself and its office bearers and also a collection of images for teaching and demonstration. The web site is managed by Andrew Downie of the Victoria Infirmary, Glasgow.

At the time of writing, a joint millennium meeting with the Royal College of Radiologists has been organised and will take place in Edinburgh in March 2000.

After more than half a century the Society, with a membership of over 300, including several overseas and honorary members, anticipates continuing its special role in furthering radiology in Scotland.

8

Current Resources

Diagnostic Radiology

In 1998 the Standing Scottish Committee of the Royal College of Radiologists sent out a comprehensive questionnaire to the clinical directors of all radiology departments in Scotland. Its aims were:

1. To examine the staffing, workload, service provision and equipment base in all Scottish departments of clinical radiology.
2. To extrapolate levels of manpower and equipment resources necessary for maintenance of service provision over the next 10 years.
3. To form recommendations for clinical radiology to ensure consistent patient care of high quality.

31 out of 33 teaching and district general hospitals responded to the survey, allowing a national baseline profile of manpower, workload and equipment to be established.

The survey was justified by the following:

1. There was an accepted long standing shortage of consultant radiologists in Scotland as evidenced by unfilled posts. In 1998 there were 22 consultant vacancies, seven having remained unfilled for more than six months. This comprised 11.5% of the consultant radiologist establishment in Scotland. By the end of 1999 the situation had deteriorated further.
2. There had been an average annual clinical consultant expansion of 4.6% across the United Kingdom over the previous five years,

not matched by clinical radiology posts which had increased by 3.7%. This increased clinical activity had made demands on departments of clinical radiology consequent on increased bed occupancy, increased patient throughput, new day-care services and one stop clinics. In addition, new and replacement clinical consultants increase clinical activity by developing specialist skills, offering new services and introducing new techniques and work practices.

3. The ever increasing complexity and frequency of investigations, particularly MRI, CT, ultrasound and interventional radiology all lead to pressure on manpower and physical resources.

4. There was (and still is) a shortfall in Scottish National Training Numbers in clinical radiology to address the workforce shortage and to allow for future expansion in relation to clinical needs.

5. The Standing Scottish Committee had concerns, shared by the Scottish Radiology Clinical Directors Forum, regarding funding of equipment replacement and the introduction of new technologies.

A summary of the results of the survey is as follows:

31 hospitals carried out a total of 2,750,686 examinations, a frequency of 537 examinations per 1,000 0f the population. International comparison shows this number to be much lower than in other developed countries. Numbers of examinations per 1,000 of the population are over 1,400 in Japan, 1,200 in Germany, 1,000 in USA and over 800 in Portugal.

The average excess workload for consultant radiologists over the level recommended by the Royal College of Radiologists was 28%, which equates to a 48 hour week. This did not include time spent on audit, teaching, research, clinical meetings, management and continuing medical education. In particular, it did not include on call which most departments find is becoming increasingly demanding. An increase in the consultant radiology manpower base of 47.3 whole time equivalents was calculated as the minimum required to bring the workload levels to those considered acceptable for continuance of quality patient care.

The total estimated replacement value of equipment in 1998 was £142,896,245. This assumed that all equipment was replaced on a 10 year programme. Using a five year replacement programme for ultrasound and seven year replacement programmes for CT and MRI, a sum of £36,241,889 was required in addition to the previous figure. The true total of estimated replacement value was therefore £179,183,134 in 1998. This figure did not include two non-responding hospitals, room preparation and pre-installation, decommissioning, other small items such as processors, some imaging equipment held outwith radiology departments, data management systems, some gamma cameras in departments of nuclear medicine and equipment that departments did not have due to lack of funding but which they needed for service provision. As an example of this under provision, there are only 14 MRI scanners in 11 out of the 33 NHS hospitals in Scotland, probably the lowest provision in western Europe.

Taking these additional items into account, the total replacement costs were estimated to be over £200 million, with an annual replacement cost approaching £30 million. In addition, almost 40% of equipment was found to be over 10 years old and therefore due for immediate replacement. Other factors which were considered to have major impact on the provision of radiological services included: increasing sophistication of equipment, reduction of ionising radiation by the use of ultrasound and MRI where appropriate, compliance with monitoring and recording of radiation dose in accordance with ionising radiation regulations, risk management and quality control, and compliance with clinical governance and national clinical protocols and guidelines. The expected development in teleradiology and picture archiving and communications systems (PACS) also have major cost implications.

As a result of the survey the report made the following recommendations:

- There is a requirement for 47 consultant radiology posts.
- To address understaffing, job vacancies and future clinical expansion, a significant increase in the Scottish training base of specialist radiology registrars is needed.
- Training for role extension, delegation and skills mix should be instituted urgently for radiographers and other care workers,

with recognition of the demands placed on radiologists for training and supervision.

- There should be managed clinical expansion across directorates and trusts to ensure that new or replacement clinical posts have matched increases in imaging services. A planned replacement equipment programme should be in place within all trusts.
- A database or asset register should be available for all imaging departments to enable monitoring of planned equipment replacement, safety aspects of radiation dosages and compliance with relevant statutes.
- New techniques and technology should be evaluated prior to planned integration into existing services.
- The introduction of PACS should be addressed urgently as a national issue with a view to rapid implementation.

Both the national breast screening programme and the pilot site for colorectal cancer screening are beginning to report difficulties with funding and recruitment. This will adversely affect the quality of patient care. Increased recruitment and a wider training base are required for radiologists. Skills mix, computer assisted reporting, changes in work practice and funding are also under consideration to address the current problems in the breast screening programme. Similar solutions need to be considered for the colorectal cancer screening programme.

Radiotherapy and Oncology

Radiotherapy is the second most effective treatment for cancer after surgery. Approximately 70% of patients who come to radiotherapy departments receive treatment with curative intent, either by radiotherapy alone or in conjunction with surgery and chemotherapy. Of these around 50% are cured. Many of the remaining patients treated palliatively will have had an improvement in their quality of life.

Radiotherapy is a very cost effective treatment. Because each linear accelerator delivers 200,000 to 300,000 exposures in its working lifetime, the unit cost of treatment is low. In spite of a major increase in the use of cytotoxic chemotherapy, hormone therapy and immunotherapy in the last twenty years, there has been no reduction in the annual steady increase in the use of radiotherapy.

The incidence of cancer in Scotland is 4,500 per million head of population, with 50% of all cancer patients presenting in 1997 being treated by radiotherapy. The workload in terms of exposures increased by 4.6% between 1992 and 1997.

This work was carried out by 15 linear accelerators, or 2.8 per million of population. The ideal is considered to be 6 linear accelerators per 1.25 million. Broken down by district the numbers are 2.1 per million in Glasgow, 3.1 in Edinburgh, 3.6 in Aberdeen, 4.0 in Inverness and 4.4 in Dundee.

Linear accelerators should have an active life of 10 years. In Scotland in 1997, four of the 15 linear accelerators were 10 years or older; five were 6–9 years old and six were 1–5 years old. A reasonable workload for a modern linear accelerator is 20,000 exposures per year. The range of exposures per linear accelerator per year in 1997 was 16,700–30,000. Assuming a ten year life expectancy, 10% of the stock should be replaced each year. In order to keep up with increasing demand and need, a growth factor of 5% per year should be added. Any increase in equipment needs to be accompanied by appropriate increases in staffing which should include radiotherapists, radiographers, physicists an technicians.

Waiting times for radiotherapy are an indication of the availability of patient access to linear accelerators in a region. Recommended waiting times are as follows:

Patient Group	Good Practice	Maximum Acceptable Delay
A Urgent	24 hours	48 hours
B Radical	14 days	28 days
C Palliative	2 days	14 days
D Post-operative		48 days

In 1998, Edinburgh just met the maximum recommended waiting times whereas Glasgow exceeded the time with a maximum waiting time of 104 days for radical radiotherapy and 97 days for adjuvant breast radiotherapy.

The consequences of under provision are long waiting lists for radiotherapy; an inability to deliver best effective treatment and an inability to compensate for potentially fatal delays in treatment.

Extra linear accelerators and supporting staff and infrastructure are urgently needed to provide up to four linear accelerators per million of population. This means that 12 new linear accelerators are required. Since this survey was conducted, the Scottish Health Service has awarded funding for two new and six replacement accelerators. Two of these are scheduled for Glasgow, the area currently with the poorest provision.

Appendix I

Scottish Radiological Society Office Bearers

Presidents

1936–37	J S Fulton
1937–45	J B King
1946	R McWhirter
1947–49	G G Chartois
1949–51	D M Harper
1951–53	W S Shearer
1953–55	J G McWhirter
1955–57	D P Levack
1957–59	R McWhirter
1959–61	R Saffley
1961–63	W C Swanson
1963–65	S D Scott Park
1965–67	J C Davidson
1967–69	W McLeod
1969–72	A J Sangster
1972–73	D H Cummack
1973–74	J M Glennie
1974–75	S Haase
1975–76	J G Duncan
1976–77	P Aitken
1977–78	T B Brewin
1978–79	T Philp
1979–80	T N Cowie
1980–81	F Kelly
1981–82	M W M Hadley
1982–83	A A Donaldson
1983–84	J S Scott
1984–85	W S Copland

1985–86	K Wood
1986–87	E R Watson
1987–88	G R Sutherland
1988–89	A F MacDonald
1989–91	H Yosef
1991–93	W J A Gibson
1993–95	J W McNab
1995–97	A Barrett
1997–99	J F Calder
1999–	R H Corbett

Honorary Secretaries

1946	K Harper
1947–55	D P Levack
1955–59	R Saffley
1959–63	W L Munro
1963–66	J G Duncan
1966–70	S Haase
1971–74	A F MacDonald
1974–77	F Kelly
1977–80	W J A Gibson
1980–84	J S Soutar
1984–86	H Yosef
1986–89	R H Corbett
1989–92	J F Calder
1992–95	A Harnett
1995–98	A S Hollman
1998–	G M Baxter

Appendix II

Radiologists in Scotland, Present and Past, as at March 2000

Royal Infirmary, Glasgow

D E Anderson	1981-	J Macintyre	1895-1926
A Forrester	1989-	J Gilchrist	1900-1901
E L S L Leen	1995-	J R Riddell	1902-1920
J Litherland	1996-	K M Chapman	1920-1924
D H A McCarter	1996-	A B MacLean	1925-1939
F W Poon	1990-	D Macintyre	1923-1929
A W Reid	1989-	R M C Crawford	1927-1940
G H Roditi	1997-	A Balfour Black	1923-1941
I S Stewart	1981-	R A Kemp Harper	1939-1946
		M C Leishman	1941-1942
		N Klein	1942-1945
		E Timoshenko (Calder)	1942-1969
		J Z Walker	1947-1968
		A A Vickers	1944-1947
		S Haase	1950-1961
		D Raeside	1950-1978
		N J McKellar	1963-1988
		B Moule	1966-1995
		J G Duncan	1969-1987
		T D Lightbody	1969-1990
		O P Fitzgerald-Finch	1974-1976
			1978-1981
		S Yogarajah	1977-1985
		G R Sutherland	1987-1991

Western Infirmary, Glasgow

F G Adams	1971-	D J Mackintosh	1892-1920
G M Baxter	1993-	W F Sommerville	1908-1920
M D Cowan	1980-	A Hay	1908-1920
W Kincaid	1994-	J G Tomkinson	1908
N McMillan	1983-	J R Riddell	1920-1932
N Raby	1992-	J S Fulton	1933-1939
G Stenouse	1981-	S D Scott Park	1939-1967

		D Stenhouse	-1973
		T N Cowie	1954-1981
		E Barnett	1956-1986
		J K Davidson	1967-1990
		P Morley	-1993
		G T McCreath	1976-1978

Gartnavel General Hospital

R Edwards	1997-	D Stenhouse	1973-1977
J Moss	1992-	T N Cowie	1973-1981
R Vallance	1977-	A Aylmer	1973-1979
L Wilkinson	1993-		
A-M Sinclair	1999-		

Stobhill Hospital, Glasgow

F Bryden	1992-	A Balfour Black	1925-1960
H Griffiths	1999-	S Haase	1961-1977
G McCreath	1998-	A McGregor	1960-
I MacLeod	1988-	H C Anton	1963-1983
J Shand	1987-	J R M Wilson	1967-1990
M Sproule	1998-	G R Sutherland	1977-1991
R Stevens	1995-	J Negrette	1984-1993
		B Anastasi	
		S Ingram	1994-1998

Victoria Infirmary, Glasgow

J F Calder	1986-	D O McGregor	1919-1929
A C Downie	1998-	G J Wilson	1929-1946
S E G Goudie	1984-	J Innes	1946-1972
J C Lauder	1991-	C K Blum	1943-1966
I M McLaughlin	1999-	J Lawson	1953-1984
W R Pickard	1991-	H Gardner	1961-1985
		J S H Davidson	1966-1991
		M A Millar	1972-1999
		F Howie	1989-1993
		G C McInnes	1993-1997
		G McKillop	1995-1997
		R Connor	1998-2000

Southern General Hospital, Glasgow

C Campbell	1990-	R Crawford	
P Duffy	1992-	A Balfour Black	
R Johnstone	1998-	A McGregor	-1960
L Stewart	1998-	W Dempster	-1960
G D K Urquhart	1995-	J K Davidson	1960-1967
		W B James	1964-1987
		K Grossart	1961-1964
		G R Sutherland	1968-1977

D A R Robertson	1966-1998
G T McCreath	1978-1998

Institute of Neurological Sciences, Glasgow

J Battacharya	1997-	J L Steven	-1974
D M Hadley	1985-	K Grossart	1961-1992
D Kean	1994-	P Macpherson	1969-1990
E Teasdale	1979-	J Dervin	1994-1997
		J Wardlaw	1992-1994

Royal Hospital for Sick Children, Glasgow

B Fredericks	1990-	J Riddell	
J R MacKenzie	1977-	D C Suttie	1914-1953
A McLennan	1997-	S P Rawson	1953-1978
S Maroo	1998-	E M Sweet	1963-1988
A Watt	2000-	M McNair	1971-1978
		M Ziervogel	1978-1992
		A S Hollman	1988-1999
		G Wilkinson	1993-1998

Breast Screening Service, Glasgow

C Alexander	1997-	F Howie	1989-1995
C Cordiner	1990-	J Lauder	1991-1997
H M Dobson	1988-	B Dall	1990-1992
H Griffiths	1999-		
J Litherland	1996-		
N Moss	1994-		
W R Pickard	1991-		
L Wilkinson	1993-		

Specialist Registrars, Glasgow

B Alabdi	1997-
B Adlung	1997-
E Beveridge	1995-
J Ballantyne	1996-
S Ballantyne	1997-
I Britton	1995-
D Brydie	1998-
S Butler	1996-
N T Corrigan	1994-
N Dawson	1999-
D Edwards	1996-
M Elabassy	1995-
S Evans	1996-
L Foo	1998-
J Gordon	1999-
T Halliday	1996-
B Hamilton	1997-

K Hammer	1995-
J Howells	1999-
G Irwin	1998-
V Jayakrishnan	1997-
S C Jenkins	1995-
E Kalkman	1997-
S Kelly	1996-
C K Koo	1995-
S Kumar	1995-
P F Lau	1997-
A McCafferty	1997-
S Macdonald	1995-
D McNally	1997-
A Mizzi	1999-
J Morrison	1995-
G O'Neil	1997-
A Pover	1998-
S Rai	1999-
M Sambrook	1996-
A Shabani	1999-
J Walker	1999-

Beatson Oncology Centre, Glasgow

Clinical Oncology

A Armour	1999-	S Bundi
A Barrett (Prof.)	1986-	T Brewin
P Canney	1989-	K Calman
D Dodds	1996-	A Gregor
T Habeshaw	1978-	K Halnan
A Harnett	1988-	F McGurk
R Jones	1991-	A Nias
E Junor	1994-	H Porter
A McDonald	1999-	P Symonds
N O'Rourke	1997-	I McHattie
R Rampling	1987-	E Watson
N Reed	1984-	M Cowell
D Ritchie	1994-	N Russell
A G Robertson	1982-	F Kelly
M Russell	1988-	J Davidson
H Yosef	1974-	D Andrew
F Yuille	1999-	

Medical Oncology

D Dunlop	J Cassidy
J Evans	D Kerr (Professor)
S Kaye (Professor)	
C Twelves	
P Vasey	

Specialist Registrars, Clinical Oncology
F Cowie
C Featherstone
G Fraser
F Kent
R McMenemin
N Mahommed
K Turner
J Wallace

Specialist Registrars, Medical Oncology
A Anthony
S Barrett
M Eatock
C McGregor
R Glasspool
J Debono

Royal Infirmary, Edinburgh

P Allan	1983-	D Turner	1898-1925
I Beggs	1983-	J Spence	1901-1907
T Buckenham (Prof.)	1999-	W H Fowler	1901-
I Gillespie	1987-	A McKendrick	
S Ingram	1998-	J W Morison	1926-1930
A Kirkpatrick	1973-	D White	1930-1937
K McBride	1994-	A E Barclay	1936
G McInnes	1997-	R McWhirter (Prof)	1937-1946
G McKillop	1997-	J P McGibbon	1942-1952
J Murchison	1994-	W S Shearer	1946-1957
D Patel	1999-	A A Donaldson	1966-1957
I Prossor	1975-	B Young	1964-1980
D Redhead	1979-	E Samuel (Prof)	1958-1978
J Walker	1995-	T Philp	1956-1986
J Walsh	1988-	T A S Buist	1969-1985
A Wightman	1975-	M Summerling	-1979
T Fitzgerald	2000-	J G Duncan	1956-1969
		K Wood	-1968
		A Duncan	
		W Ritchie	
		J J K Best (Prof)	1979-1998
		D Kean	1983-1991
		B Muir	1984-1988
		S Chambers	1984-1999
		J Reid	1986-1996
		S Rimmer	1980-1982

Western General Hospital, Edinburgh

J P Brush	1999-	H Cummack	1947-1977
M E Chapman	1996-	W A Copland	1956-
D A Collie	1996-	A A Donaldson	1957-1987
M L Errington	1999-	D J Sinclair	1972-1975
R Gibson	1994-	G M Fraser	1968-1991
D C Grieve	1978-	J G Cruikshank	
S A Moussa	1991-	M V Merrick	1974-1999
R J Sellar	1986-	A R Wright	
A J M Stevenson	1989-		
C M Turnbull	1979-		
G T Vaughan	1971-		
J M Wardlaw	1994-		
S R Wild	1975-		

Lothian Primary Care Trust

Eastern General, Liberton, Edenhall, Roodlands, Leith, The Royal Edinburgh Astley Ainsley

R Adam	1987-	R McWhirter	1942-1947
J J K Best	1979-	H Cummack	1947
S Chambers	1999-	M Fraser	-1978
H L McDonald	1987-	D Grieve	
		N Thomson	-1987
		N Speirs	

The Royal Edinburgh Hospital for Sick Children

G M A Hendry	1977-	H Rainy	1897-1901
S Mackenzie	1990-	J Spence	1907-1929
M Mc Phillips	1995-	G Allan	1929-1956
G Wilkinson	1998-	W McLeod	1947-1976
		D J Sinclair	1972-1975
		S R Wild	1975-1986

Breast Screening, Edinburgh

M E Chapman	1997-
A E Kirkpatrick	1988-
B B Muir	1988-
J S Walsh	1988-

J Murray (Staff grade physician)

Specialist Registrars, Edinburgh

J Anderson
A Crean
F Ewing
F Farquarson
L Ferrando
S Glancy

S Guy
S Jackson
M Lewinski
I Masani
A Matthews
J O'Neill
F Paterson
F Perks
E Ramage
R Ramroop
C Rowlands
D Summers
S Young
N Humphries, Clinical Lecturer

Clinical Oncology, Western General Hospital, Edinburgh

Clinical Oncologists

V J Cowie	1987-	R McWhirter (Prof.)	1937-1970
A Gregor	1983-	W M Court Brown	
G Howard	1987-	K MacKenzie	
I H Kunkler	1988-	G Newaishy	
F Little	1988-	M Douglas	
D McLaren	1988-	J F G Pearson	
C McLean	1996-	J Newall	
R H McDougall	1986-	J McLelland	
L Matheson	1990-	G Ritchie	
A Price (Prof.)	1996-	J Orr	
		A Langlands	
		S Arnott	
		W Duncan (Prof.)	-1995
		W McKillop (Prof.)	
		A Rodgers	
		S Ludgate	

Medical Oncologists
D Cameron
H Gabra
D Jodrell
R C F Leonard
M McKean
J F Smyth (Prof.)

Specialist Registrars
R Camidge
R Casasola
M Dahale

A Elliot
R Ellis
S Erridge
C Millwater
P Niblock

St John's Hospital at Howden, Livingston

P S Bailey	1994-	R Saffley	1947-1974
C J Beveridge	1999-	K Wood	1968-1993
I Parker	1981-	A Mackintosh	1974-1983
L Smart	1983-	A Duncan	1979-1980
		M E Chapman	1994-1996
		T Fitzgerald	1997-2000

Borders General Hospital, Melrose

D J Hardwick	1984-	S McCall Smith	1972-1982
H A McRitchie	1996-	I Houston	1976-1996
A J Pearson	1988-		
J H Reid	1996-		
H Shannon	1997-		

Aberdeen

Royal Infirmary

A P Bayliss	1975-	J Levack	1896-1931
M Brooks	1998-	M Connon	1931-1933
H E Deans	1986-	D P Levack	1933-
K Duncan	1996-	J Blewett	1935-
F J Gilbert (Prof.)	1989-	J Innes	1942-1946
L Gomersall	1995-	A Bain	1946-1947
J K Hussey	1981-	R McKail	
D McAteer	1999-	A Stewart	
A Murray	1995-	G Mavor	
G Needham (Prof.)	1989-	L A Gillanders	1958-1988
O J Robb	1992-	P Ward	1963-1991
E M Robertson	1982-	J Palmer	1964-1967
A P Thorpe	1997-	A F MacDonald	1964-1993
F Wallis	1998-	R Mahaffy	1965-1995
J Weir (Prof.)	1975-	J Allan	-1978
S Yule	1999-	J Cantley	-1981
		F W Smith	1979-1997
		J F Calder	1980-1986

Royal Aberdeen Children's Hospital

E J Stockdale	1980-

Woodend Hospital

A Thomson	1995-
F W Smith	1997-

Specialist Registrars
B Bleakeney
R Burgul
V Duddalwar
G Gilpin
G Iyengar
P Keston
M Kumaravel
L Kurban
S Olsen
A Seth
I Smith

Radiotherapy and Oncology

J D Bissett	1994-	E Ridley	1950-
D C Hurman	1988-	I Kirby	-1978
T K Sarkar	1976-	K Bartlett	1980-1994

Specialist Registrar
A G Macdonald

Dr Gray's Hospital, Elgin

J Addison	1994-	A Simpson	1973-1994
K Brown	1990-		

Tayside

Ninewells Hospital, Dundee and formerly Dundee Royal Infirmary

R Cameron	1996-	G Pirie	1896-1925
A M Cook	1989-	G Milln	1913-1945
R I Doull	1996-	Dr Grant	-1947
J G Houston	1995-	T S Sprunt	1940s
A S McCulloch	1990-	Dr Fleming	1940s
D McLean	1993-	C Pickard	1952-1978
G Main	1995-	G Howie	1960-1989
M J Nimmo	1990-	D Dewar	-1972
J Rehman	1999-	J Soutar	
D G Sadler	1999-	D J Sinclair	1975-199?
J W Shaw	1977-	F Fletcher	1964-1996
D J Sheppard	1999-	J W McNab	1978-1998
T W Taylor	1994-	J Begg	1981-1997
C M Walker	1990-	A Thomson	1987-1995
		K Hasan	-1998
		J Ferguson	

Royal Victoria Hospital
J Begg　　　　　　1997-

Specialist Registrar
J Anderson
J Charon

Radiotherapy and Oncology

S N Das	1977-	C Swanson	1946-
J A Dewar	1986-	J Riley	1948-
A J Munro (Prof.)	1997-	J S Scott	1975-1987
P M Windsor	1987-	J Lindsay	
		R H McDougall	1982-1986

Perth Royal Infirmary

J Flinn	1994-	A Robertson	1945-
K Fowler	1995-	J McLeod	1963-
P Gamble	1984-	D Ritchie	1963-
S McClelland	1998-	J Miekle	1963-
R Murray	1981-		
R Pearson	1999-		

Stracathro and Arbroath

J Tainsh	1986-	A Elektrovitch	1940-1956
		Dr White	1956-1957
		R J C Campbell	1957-1968
		D H Sutherland	1964-
		W J A Gibson	1968-1999
		S Sutton	1984-1986
		S S Hamid	1995-1997

Raigmore Hospital, Inverness

G Aitken	1984-	J C Tainsh	1930s
D Goff	1985-	Dr Gottlieb	1940s
P Hendry	1990-	A Bain	1947-1960s
A McLeod	1999-	J C Wood	1947-
D Nichols	1986-	J Sangster	1950-1970s
A Todd	1990-	H Innes	1955-1986
F R Williams	1977-	M W M Hadley	1960-1984
R McKay	1964-		

Radiotherapy and Oncology

M H Elia	1983-	K A Mackenzie	1962-1977
D Whillis	1991-	G Jardine	1977-1982

Western Isles
I Riach　　　　　　1990-

Fife

Queen Margaret Hospital, Dunfermline

A Gilchrist	1996-	M Errington	1996-1999
A W Duncan	1999-	M Fleet	1997-1999
K A Jamieson	1999-		
H M Ireland	1996-		
M Walker	1983-		

Victoria Hospital, Kirkcaldy / Dunfermline & Kirkcaldy

C Clark	1997-	P Aitken	1947-1982
C Hendry	1973-	D R Maitland	1953-1966
W Reid	1988-	F M Leetion	1963-1969
D Smith	1973-	A A Marr	1966-1988
		A Dick	1966-1987
		A Dumbreck	1971-1996
		J R MacKenzie	1977-1979
		I J F Morle	1981-1984
		K Jawad	1982-1997
		R I Doull	1985-1996
		R C P Cameron	1986-1996
		T Fitzgerald	1987-1997
		D F McLean	1993-1997
		P McAndrew	1997-1998
		D Foulner	1997-2000

Stirling Royal Infirmary

H Cunningham	1978-	M Ziervogel	1976-1978
D Glen	1991-	S Miller	1975-1980
P McDermott	1983-	A Gilchrist	1989-1990
		S Maroo	1996-1998

Falkirk and District Royal Infirmary
Stirling and Falkirk

J E Barry	1990-	G J Wilson	-1929
A J Byrne	1970-	F O Brown	1959-1987
		M Fraser	
		R Cuthbert	-1967
		J S Brown	1967-1993
		B O'Sullivan	1969-1975
		D Harper	
		D Roxburgh	1984-1999
		S L Stewart	1995-1998

Hairmyres Hospital, East Kilbride

R Connor	1986-1998	J McWhirter	1939-1940
	2000-	J Hurrel	-1944

R H Corbett	1976-	R McKail	1944-1950
F Gardner	1985-	J Donald	1950-1951
F Howie	1994-	W Monroe	1951-
A McCallum	1996-	J Z Walker	1952-1964
S Millar	1985-	M Strathern	1964-1966
F Mohsen	1983-	W M Campbell	1968-1980s
C Murch	1998-	R Freeland	1966-1977
R Weir	1977-	I Gray-Thomas	1967-1979
		W Mowatt	1971-1977

Law Hospital, Carluke

D Alcorn	1997-	M Leach	Pre1962
M Callaghan	1994-	W Dempster	1960-1980s
M El-Sayed	1984-	W Mowatt	1971-1997
M Fleet	1999-	J Bell	1972-1993
B Macpherson	1995-	E J McKay	1977-1996
S Reid	1996-	D K Pattnaik	1977-1996
J Roberts	1988-	G Urquhart	1990-1995
		A Robertson	1993-1998

Monklands Hospital, Airdrie

G Dewar	1999-	R Freeland	1977-1982
J Guse	1993-	W Mowatt	1977-1998
M J Gronski	1998-	J A Johnstone	1978-1999
R M Holden	1979-		
K Hughes	1982-		
K Wallers	1984-		

Royal Alexandra Hospital Paisley

C Adams	1999-	Dr Stirling	-1973
C Alexander	1984-	A Stevenson	-1977
L Cram	1985-	J McLean	-1984
M-L Davies	1991-	J McCavena	-1984
J J Negrette	1993-	J G Paterson	-1998
M J Stevenson	1987-		
A Wallace	1997-		

Inverclyde Royal Hospital, Greenock

F Kelly	1988-	M Strathern	1966-1993
A Ramsay	1993-	J Galloway	1975-1988
R Shaw	1993-		
P Walsh	1989-		

Vale of Leven Hospital, Alexandria

I McGlinchey	1997-	T N Cowie	1954-1963
		B McKee	1963-1985
		J Galloway	1988-1985
		I Jackson	1985-1995

| | | J Zachary | 1996-1997 |
| | | P Gill | 1997-1998 |

Lorne and Islands Hospital, Oban

| J Galloway | 1996- |
| P J Lane | 1998- |

Crosshouse Hospital, Kilmarnock

P Crumlish	1976-	Dr McCrorie	
M Dean	1990-	R Crawford	
E L S Lindsay	1986-	W Monroe	
G McLaughlin	1995-	D Urquhart	
M A H McMillan	1979-	J Smith	1971-1994
D Rawlings	1990-	B Stanton	1978-1999

The Ayr Hospital

M Ablett	1998-	Dr Mackie	-1969
D Chanock	1998-	B Reid	-1971
S Cooper	1998-	M Greenhill	1969-1998
K N A Osborne	1994-	D Russell	1973-1997
A Robertson	1998-	H Cunningham	1975-1978
		G McLaughlin	1986-1995
		C Murch	1990-1998
		D Rawlings	1990-1994

Dumfries and Galloway Royal Infirmary

D Hill	1986-	J McWhirter	1947-1961
P Kelly	1999-	L Frain -Bell	1961-1986
P Law	1992-	S McCall Smith	1961-1972
G Watson	1982-	D E A Dewar	1972-1984
		D Jones	1974-1998

Garrick Hospital, Stranraer

| | | J Richard (GP) | 1939-1973 |
| | | R Scott (GP) | 1973- |

Bibliography

The New Electrical Pavilion at the Glasgow Royal Infirmary.
John Macintyre
The Glasgow Medical Journal vol. LXVIII no.3, 162–268, 1902

John Macintyre in Men of The Day. A Monthly Biographical
Journal.
Ludensian Press. London. 1903

New Apparatus for The Production of X-Rays and High
Frequency Currents.
John Macintyre
The Glasgow Medical Journal vol. LXII no.4, 269–279, 1904

The Birth of Radiography in Scotland.
John Scott
Radiography vol. 17, 46–49, 1951

Nova et Vetera. An Early Radiologist (John Macintyre)
British Medical Journal 819, 1957

John Macintyre. Pioneer Radiologist.
Surgo (The University of Glasgow) 119–126 Whitsun 1958

Man Who Showed (John Macintyre)
Andrew Young
The Herald, March 23, 1996

The Western Infirmary 1874–1974
Loudon McQueen and Archibald B Kerr
John Horn. Glasgow and London. 1974

Forty Years of Obstetric Ultrasound 1957–1997: From A-Scope to Three Dimensions
Margaret B McNay and John E E Fleming
Ultrasound in Medicine and Biology vol. 25, no. 1, 3–56, 1999
World Federation for Ultrasound in Medicine and Biology

Investigation of abdominal masses by pulsed ultrasound.
Donald I, McVicar J, Brown T G.
The Lancet 1: 1188–1195; 1958

The History of Glasgow Royal Infirmary 1794–1994
Jacqueline Jenkinson, Michael Moss and Iain Russell
Glasgow Royal Infirmary NHS Trust
Harper Collins. Glasgow 1994

Board of Management for Glasgow Royal Infirmary and Associated Hospitals.
Report 1968–69

Stobhill Hospital. The First Seventy Years
Oliver M Watt
The University Press. Glasgow 1971

The Victoria Infirmary of Glasgow 1890–1948
Ian Murray
C L Wright. Glasgow 1967

The Victoria Infirmary of Glasgow 1890–1990
S D Slater and D A Dow
Victoria Infirmary Centenary Committee 1990

Institute of Neurological Sciences, Glasgow
Southern General Hospital
Board of Management of Glasgow South-Western Hospitals 1972

Institute of Neurological Sciences. 1970–1995. 25 Years at the Southern General Hospital
Southern General Hospital, Glasgow 1995

The Yorkhill Story
Edna Robertson
The Board of Management for Yorkhill and Associated Hospitals
Glasgow 1972

Glasgow's X-Ray Campaign Against Tuberculosis
Glasgow Corporation 1957

Working Group on Breast Cancer Screening. Report to the
Health Ministers of England, Wales Scotland and Northern
Ireland
Forrest A P M, Chairman
HMSO London 1986

Ovarian Oblation in Breast Cancer, 1896 to 1998: milestones
along hierarchy of evidence from case report to Cochrane
review
Michael J Clarke
British Medical Journal, 317: 1246–8, 1998

The Story of a Great Hospital
The Royal Infirmary of Edinburgh. 1729–1929
A Logan Turner
Oliver and Boyd. Edinburgh and London 1937

The Royal Infirmary of Edinburgh 1929–1979
E F Catford
Scottish Academic Press. Edinburgh 1984

A History of the Western General Hospital
Martin Eastwood and Anne Jenkinson
John Donald. Edinburgh 1995

The Royal Edinburgh Hospital for Sick Children. 1860–1960
Douglas Guthrie
E & S Livingstone. Edinburgh and London 1960

A Beacon in Our Town. The Story of Leith Hospital
Christine Hoy
Spectrum. Livingston 1988

Leith Hospital 1948–1988
David H A Boyd
Scottish Academic Press, Edinburgh 1990

The Bangour Story
W F Hendrie and D A D Mcleod
The Mercat Press. Edinburgh 1991

Aberdeen Royal Infirmary
The People's Hospital of the North-East
Iain D Levack and H A F Dudley
Balliere Tindall. London 1992

The Story of X-Rays — Dundee Connections
Medical History Museum. Exhibition 4
Ninewells Hospital and Medical School, Dundee. 1991

Hairmyres. The History of the Hospital
Allan Campbell
Lanarkshire Health Board. 1994

The Greenock Infirmary. 1806–1968
John Ferrier.
Greenock and District Hospitals Board of Management.
1968

The Invisible Light
A M K Thomas
Blackwell Science. Oxford 1995

Röntgen's Rays and His Scottish Disciples
Jean M Guy
Haldane Tait Lecture
The Scottish Society of the History of Medicine. 14–22. Session
1994–95 & 1995–96

The Röntgen Centenary
L W Fleming
Scottish Medical Journal. 40: 153–155, 1995

Workload, Workforce and Equipment in Departments of Clinical
Radiology in Scotland
Board of theFaculty of Clinical Radiology
The Royal College of Radiologists, London. 1999

Equipment, Workload and Staffing for Radiotherapy in Scotland
1992–1997
Board of the Faculty of Clinical Oncology
Royal College of Radiologists, London. 2000

Obituaries

Sir James McKenzie Davidson
Archives of Radiology and Electrotherapy. Vol. XXIII, No.11,
no. 225, 337–340, 1918–19

William Ironside Bruce
British Medical Journal. 481, 26th March 1921

John Macintyre
The Lancet. 1052, 17th Nov. 1928

Dawson Turner
British Journal of Radiology. Vol. 2, 330, 1929

James Robertson Riddell
The Lancet. 49, 6th July 1935

James Robertson Riddell
British Medical Journal. 90–91, 13th July 1935

J P McGibbon
British Medical Journal. 1030, 10th May 1952

J S Fulton
British Medical Journal. 639–40, 11th March 1967

James Z Walker
British Medical Journal. 3; 504, 24th August 1968

Thomas Alexander Buist
Clinical Radiology. 37; 123–125, 1986

Ian Donald
Clinical Radiology. 37; 7, 1988

Andrew Alexander Donaldson
Clinical Radiology. 37; 7–8, 1988

Robert McWhirter
The Scotsman. 7th November 1994

Robert McWhirter
British Medical Journal. Vol. 310; 54, 1995

Thomas Philp
Clinical Radiology. 50; 353, 1995

David Hunter Cummack
Clinical Radiology. 51; 529–530, 1996

Eric Samuel
The Scotsman. 24th Sept. 1997

Eric Samuel
Clinical Radiology. 52; 966–967, 1997

Irene Jackson
The Herald. 13th July 1999

Andrew Dick
British Medical Journal. Vol. 319; 156, 1999

Anne Sheila Dutton (Hollman)
The Herald. 4th December 1999

Anne Sheila Dutton (Hollman)
British Medical Journal. Vol. 320; 189, 2000

Index

Aberdeen 5, 8, 11, 14, 27, 40, 41, 51, **55–64**
  City Hospital 58
  Royal Aberdeen Children's Hospital 60
Aberdeen Evening Express 59
Aberdeen Royal Infirmary 5, 23, **56–61**, **62–64**
Aberdeen University 23, **59–60**, 63, 86
Adam, Richard 48
Adams, Calum 77
Adams, Frederick 18, 19
Addison, John 62
Aitken, George 71
Aitken, Peter 72
Albanian 86
Alcorn, Desmond 76
Alexander, Carole 77
Alexander, Dr 61
Allan, Grant 47
Allan, Michael 58
Allan, Paul 21, 42
American Red Cross 49
ANCHOR 64
Anderson, Dorothy 13
Anderson, Lady Mary 52

M D Anderson Cancer Center 67
Angiography 18, 23, 26, 27, 40, 57, 67, 70, 78, 81
Anton, Craigie 22
Arbroath 68
Argyle and Clyde 76–78
Argyll, Duchess of 32
Astley Ainsley Hospital 47
Auld, John Leckie 84
Australia 78
Aylmer, Albert 22
Ayr 79
Ayr County Hospital 79
Ayr Hospital 79
Ayrshire 78–79

Babcock and Wilcox 20
Bailey, Peter 50
Bain, Alexander 57, 70
Ballantrae 37
Ballochmyle Hospital 79
Banff 58
Bangour Hospital 49
Bank of Scotland 52
Barclay, Alfred E 37, 38, 53
Barnett, Ellis 18, 21, 59
Barrett, Ann 33

Barry, Jo 73
Bauer Tube 49
Baxter, Grant 19, 21, 42
Bayliss, A P 59
Beatson Institute 33
Beatson Oncology Centre 34
Beatson, Sir George 32
Beechmount 52, 53
Beggs, Ian 42
Belfast 40
Bell, Clifford T 56
Bell, John 56
Belvidere Hospital 33, 34
Bessent, Rodney 15
Best, Jonathan 40, 49
Beveridge, Carolyn 50
bismuth meal 16
Black, Alan Balfour 11, 22, 25
Blackwood, Matthew 77
Blewett, John 56, 57, 61, 80, 81
Blum, Karel 24
Blumgart, Leslie 12
Blythswood, Lord 1, 3
Borders 45, 50, 55
Borders General Hospital 42, 50
Bottomley, J T 1, 3
breast cancer 54, 55 (see also screening)
Brechin 67
Brewin, Thurston 33
Bridge of Earn Hospital 67
Briggs, Sister 61
Bristol Myers 85
Britain 3, 5, 43
British 30, 39, 81
British Institute of Radiology 39, 74, 82, 83, 86

British Laryngological, Rhinological and Otological Association 2
British Red Cross Society 37
British Society of Neuroradiologists 46
Brown, Kenneth 62
Brown, Tom 20
Browne, J Nixon 30
Bruce, William Ironside 8
Bryden, Fiona 22
Buckenham, Tim 42
Buist, T A S 41, 42
Burrell, Lady 32

Calder, John 24, 59
Calman, Sir Kenneth 33
Cambridge 23, 37, 39
Cameron, Mr 21
Campbell, Colin 26
Campbell, Robert 68
Campbell, William 75
Canada 78
Cancer Control Organisation 53
Cancer Relief McMillan Fund 55
Cancer Research Campaign 34
Canniesburn Hospital 13
Cape Town 20
Cardiff 39
Carnegie, Andrew 3, 72
Carnegie, Louise 71
Castle Douglas 80
Chambers, Sarah, 49
Chapman, Katherine 50, 51
Chapman, Melanie 11
Chief Medical Officer 33, 83
Christie Hospital 23, 37
cine radiography 3, 57

Citrin, Denis 15
City Hospital, Aberdeen 58
City Hospital, Edinburgh
    42, 48
Cleon 44
Clinical Nurosciences 45–46
Clinical Population and
    Cytogenetics Unit 54
cobalt 33, 63, 65, 70
computer 25
Connor, Rachel 75
Conon, Middleton, 56
Conrad, Joseph 2
contrast media 67
Coolidge Tube 16, 79
Copland, William A 43
Corbett, Robert 74
Cornwall 20
Corporation Hospitals 42, 47
Court Brown, William A 54,
    84
Cowan, Michael 19
Cowie, Tom 18, 77–78
Cowie, Valerie 55
Cox's Vacuum Tube 9
Cram, Lester 11, 25, 78
Crawford, Robert 11, 25, 78
Cresswell Maternity Hospital
    80
Crichton Mental Hospital 80
Crosshouse Hospital 11, 78
Cruikshank, John 44, 62
Crumlish, Patrick 79
CT 13, 18, 19, 22, 24, 26,
    27, 29, 40, 44, 46, 50,
    58, 62, 66, 71, 74–75,
    77, 79, 81, 88
Culduthel Isolation Hospital
    69
Cummack, Hunter 42, 48, 85

Cunningham, Hazel 73
Curie, Marie 67
Curie Foundation 32
Currie, Sir Alexander 86
Cyprus 86
Cyprus Radiological Society 86

Dalbeattie 80
Dalhousie University 4
Daliburgh Hospital 71
Das, Sachi 65
Davidson, J C 84
Davidson, J Stuart H 24, 25
Davidson, James Mackenzie
    5, 56
Davidson, John Knight 18,
    19, 25
Davies, Marie-Louise 77
Deaconess Hospital 47
Dean's Vacuum Tube 9
Dempster, William 25, 75–76
Department of Health 50,
    83
Dewar, Derrick 66, 81
Dewar, Gordon 76
Dewar, John 66
Diasonograph 20, 41
Dick, Andrew 72
Dingwall 70
Diploma in Radiology 17
Dobson, Hilary 31
Donald, Ian 20–21
Donald, J 73
Donaldson, Andrew
    Alexander 41, **44–46**, 58
Doppler 14
Dot, Norman 44, 49
Douglas, John 75
Douglas, Mary 54
Downie, Andrew 24, 86

Duffy, Paul 26
Dumbarton 78
Dumfries Academy 42
Dumfries and Galloway 55,
    79–81
Dumfries and Galloway
    Royal Infirmay 79–81, 83
Duncan, Andrew 49
Duncan, James G 13, 41
Duncan, William 55
Dundee 5–7, 24, 31, 47, 51,
    65–67
    Maryfield Hospital 66
    Ninewells Hospital **66–67**
Dundee Royal Infirmary 5,
    6, **65–67**
Dunfermline 71–72
Dunfermline and West Fife
    Hospital 72
Dunfermline Cottage
    Hospital 71
Duntocher Hospital 78

East Fortune Hospital 48
East Kilbride 73–75
Eastern General Hospital 47
Eddison, Thomas 4
Edenhall Hospital 47
Edinburgh 4, 5, 7, 13, 16,
    18, 20, 22, 24, 25, 26,
    27, 31, **35–49**, **50–55**,
    62, 63, 65, 70
Edinburgh Academy 38
Edinburgh Medico-
    Chirurgical Society 4
Edinburgh Royal Infirmary
    7, 12, **35–42**, 43, 44, 46,
    52–54
Edinburgh University 37,
    38, 40, 42, 50, 52, 53

education 25, 29, 38, 44, 46,
    56, 57, 73, 76, 80
Edward, John Hall 7
Edwards, Richard 19
Egyptian Society of
    Radiology and Nuclear
    Medicine 86
electrical department 3, 6,
    35, 69
Electrovich, Adam 67–68
Elgin 61–62
Elia, Mumtaz 70
El-Sayed, Mohammed 76
Elscint 45, 58
EMI 20, 26, 66, 67
England 86
ERCP 12, 24, 44
Errington, Martin 45
European Association of
    Radiologists 84
European Society of
    Paediatric Radiologists 28
Evans, W G 63
Eye Infirmary 10

Faculty of Medicine 14
Faculty of Radiologists 11,
    17, 40, 43, 53, 80, 83
Falkirk 72, 73
Falkirk and District Royal
    Infirmary 23, 29, **72–73**
Fettes College 20
Fife 45, 55, **71–72**, 74
Fitzgerald Finch, Patrick 13
Fitzgerald, Tom 50
Flatman, Gerald 33
Fleet, Mustafa 76
Fleming, Dr 65
Fletcher, Frank 66
Flinn, Janet 67

Fogelman, Ignac 15
Forbes Chair of Medical
    Radiology 38, 40, 53
Foresterhill **56–57**, 58, 60,
    63, 64, 72, 73, 85
Forrest, Patrick 31–50
Forrester, Alastair 14
Fort William 70
Forth Valley 72–73
Fowler, Alexander Coutts 61
Fowler, Kenneth 67
Fowler, William Hope 7, 35,
    36
Frain-Bell, Lockhart 80
Fraser Foundation 16
Fraser, Martin 44, 48
Fraser, Miss 61
Fredericks, Briony 29
Freeland, Robin 74, 76
Fulton, J Struthers 16, 17

Galashiels 50, 80
Galbraith, Sam 22
Galloway 79–81
Galloway, John 77, 78
Gamble, Peter 67
gamma camera 15, 29, 44,
    50
gamma rays 33
Gardner, Fiona 75
Gardner, Harry 11, 24, 25
Garrick Hospital 80
Gartnavel General Hospital
    18, 22, 34
Gateside Hospital 77
General Medical Council 57
general practitioners 78, 80
German 73, 80
Germany 6, 88
Gibson, Roderick 46

Gibson, William 68
Gilbert, Fiona 11, 60
Gillanders, Lewis A 57, 59
Gillespie, Ian 42
Glasgow 1, 3, 4, **9–34**, 59,
    62–64, 67, 91, 92
Glasgow Academy 18
Glasgow City Chambers 86
Glasgow Corporation 9, 11,
    30
Glasgow Ear, Nose and
    Throat Hospital 33
Glasgow Royal Cancer
    Hospital 32, 33
Glasgow Royal Hospital for
    Sick Children 10, 20, **28–
    29**
Glasgow Royal Infirmary 2,
    3, **9–15**, 16, 22, 24, 32,
    33, 41, 44, 74, 76
Glasgow Royal Maternity
    Hospital 20, 23, 34
Glasgow School of Art 84
Glasgow University 2, 3, 12,
    14, 15, 17, 23, 24, 33
Gleneagles 46, 84
Glyn Evans lecturer 40
Goff, David 71
Gogarburn Hospital 48
Gold Medal 54
Golspie 70
Gotlieb, Dr 69
Goudie, Stella 24
Gourock 77
Govan Poor House 25
Grampian Health Board 60
Grant, Dr 65
Gray, Harry 15
Gray-Thomas, Isobel 74
Greenhill, Michael 79

Greenock 33, 74, 76, 77
Greenock Royal Infirmary 37
Gregor, Anna 55
Greig, William 15
Grieve, Douglas 44, 48
Griffith, Harry 56, 63
Gronski, Michael 76
Grossart, Kenneth 25, 26, 27
Guse, Julian 76
Guy's Hospital 24

Haase, Sidney 12, 22
Hadley, Donald M 11, 27
Hadley, M W M 11, 70–71
Hairmyres Hospital 11, 73
Halnan, Keith 33, 85
Hamburg memorial 7
Hamburg, St George's Radiotherapy Hospital 7
Hammersmith Hospital 14
Hardwick, David 50
Harper, Robert Kemp 11
Hay, Archibald 16
Health Acts 85
Heathfield Hospital 79
Hendry, Michael 47
Hendry, Peter 71
Hess, Rudolf 42
Highland **69–71**, 85
Hill, David 81
Hodston, Sir James 36
Holden, Ruth 76
Holland, Thurston 7
Hollman, Anne 29
Holt Radium Institute 17, 53
Hooper, Lesley 15
Houston, Graham 67
Houston, Iain 50

Howard, Grahame 55
Howie, Fiona 11, 75
Howie, George 66
human genome 54
Hunterian Professor 40
Hurrel, J 73
Hussey, Jefferey K 59, 61
Hutcheon, Andrew 14
Hutchison, James 59

Ingram, Susan 22, 44
Innes, John 23, 57
Institute of Neurological Sciences 11, 12, 13, **26–28**
Institute of Radiotherapeutics and Oncology 33
Inverclyde Royal Hospital 77
Inverness 31, 51, 57, 58, **69–71**
Ireland 86
Irvine 31, 51
Irvine, Sir Henry 2
isotope scanner 15

Jackson, Irene 78
James, Wilson B 25, 26, 78
Japan 20, 41, 88
Jardine, George 70
Johnstone, Edward 69
Johnstone, J 73, 74
Johnstone, James 76
Johnstone, Robert 26
Jones, David 81

Kelly, Peter 77
Kelvin, Lord 1, 2, 3, 4, 20
Kelvin-Hughes 20
Kenya Association of Radiologists 86

Kenya(n) 29, 86
Killearn Hospital 26
Kilmarnock 78
Kincaid, Wilma 19
King George V 32
King, J B 83
King's College Hospital 28, 36
Kirby, Ian 64
Kirkcaldy 72
Kirkcaldy Cottage Hospital 72
Kirkcudbright 42, 80
Kirkgunzeon 42
Kirkpatrick, Alastair 41, 42, 51
Klein, Robert 11
Knightswood Hospital 22
Knox, Robert 36
Kodak 81, 85
Krakow University 67
Kretz 41
Kuenen, Johannes 6
Kunkler, Ian 55

Lanarkshire 73–76
Langholm 80
Langlands, Allan 54
Larkfield Hospital 77
Laser Line 58
Lauder, Jean 25
Law Hospital 11, 25, **75–76**
Law, Penny 81
Lawson, John 24
Leach, Matthew 75
Leen, Eddie 14
Leishman, M C 11
Leith Hospital 47, 48
Levack, David P 56–57, 61, 62, 80

Levack, John 56, 62
Liberton Hospital 47
Lightbody, Derek 13
Lincolnshire Cancer Organisation 12
Lindsay, D W 39
Lindsay, Elspeth 11
linear accelerator 33, 64, 91–92
Litherland, Janet 14
Little, Felicity 55
Liverpool 4, 7, 17, 19
Livingstone, David 2
London 3, 5, 8, 14, 20, 24, 28, 32, 36, 37, 39, 40, 44, 53
Lorne and Islands Hospital 78
Lothian Health Board 55
Lothian Primary Care Trust 47
Lothians 45, 47, 55
Lothians University Hospitals 44

M & D Technology 59
Macalister Wiggin tube 49
Macdonald, Alexander F 57, 58
Macintyre, Donald 2
Macintyre, Donald Livingstone 11
Macintyre, John **2–4**, **9–11**, 16, 20
Macintyre, Margaret 2
Mack, Alistair 24
Mackenzie Davidson interrupter 9
Mackenzie Davidson localiser 5

MacKenzie, J Ruth 29
Mackenzie, Stephanie 47
Mackie, Dr 79
Mackintosh, Donald J 15, 21
Maclean, Bruce 11
MacLennan, Alexander 29
Macpherson, Barbara 11, 76
Macpherson, Peter 11, 26
Madras College 15
Mahaffy, Ronald 40, 58, 59
Mailer, Robert 23
Major, John 79
Mallard, John 59
mammography 15, 31, 51, 58, 67, 70
Manchester 17, 23, 37, 38, 41
Marischal College 63
Maroo, Sanjay 29
martyrs 4, 7–8, 36, 46
Matheson, Lillian 55
Mavor and Coulson 9
Mavor, George 57
Mayo Clinic 23, 37
McBride, Keiron 42
McCall-Smith, Sam 50, 80
McCallum, Angela 75
McCarter, Douglas 14
McClelland, Suzanne 67
McCreath, Gina 22, 26
McCrorie, Dr 78
McDermot, Peter 73
McDonald, H L 48
McDougal, Ross 15
McDougall, Hugh 55, 65
McFadyean, Dr 63, 69
McGibbon, John Paton 38, 39, 84
McGirr, Edward 14
McGlinchey, Ian 78

McGregor, Agnes 22, 25
McGregor, Duncan O 23
McGregor, Sir Alexander 74
McInnes, George 24, 41
McKail, Robert 57, 60, 73
McKay, Edward J 76
McKee, Ben 78
McKellar, Nimmo 12
McKendrick, Archibald 7, 35
McKenzie, Kenneth 70
McKillop, Graham 25, 29, 31
McKillop, James 15
McKillop, William 55
McKintosh, Alastair 49
McLean, Catriona 55
McLean, J 77
McLelland, James 54
McLeod, Andrew 71
McLeod, Ian 22
McLeod, John 67
McLeod, William 47
McMillan, Morag 79
McMillan, Nigel 19
McNab, Winton 66
McNair, Sister 73, 74
McNicol, George 60
McPhillips, Maeve 47
McRitchie, Hamish 50
McRobert lecturer 63
McRobert, Georgina 62
McVicar, John 20
McWhirter, John 73, 79, 83
McWhirter, Robert 37, 38, 40, 48, 52–54, 82, 83
Mearnskirk Hospital 24
medical electricians 4, 35, 36
Medical Research Council 27, 54
Meek, David 13

megavoltage x-rays 33
Melba, Dame Nellie 2
Merchants' House 22
Merrick, Malcolm 44–45, 67
Metalix tube 61
Metropolitan-Vickers 38, 53
Middlemiss, Howard 85
Middlesex Hospital 32, 39, 40
Millan, Bruce 26
Millar, Mary 24, 35
Millar, Sam 74
Milln, George 65
Milton Keynes 13
Mohsen, Fatma 74
Mombasa 86
Monklands Hospital 74, 76
Monroe, William 73, 74
Morison, J Woodburn 37
Morley, Patricia 21, 59
Moss, Jonathan 19
Moule, Brian 12, 13
Mousewald 79
Mowatt, William 75, 76
MRI 14, 19, 26, 27, 29, 40, 42, 46, 47, 59, 60, 67, 72, 79, 88, 89
Muir, B B 42, 51
Muirhead Professor 14, 15
Mull of Galloway 80
Munro, Alastair 66
Murch, Clifford 75
Murison, C A 53
Murray, Allison 60
Murray, Hugh 32
Murray, Jean 52
Murray, Provan 14
Murray, Richard 67
Murray, Robert Milne 4
Murrayfield Hospital 66

Nairn 70
Nairn, Michael B 72
National Health Service 12, 17, 18, 33, 42, 47, 57, 58, 61, 70, 79, 82, 83, 84, 85
National Radium Commission 52, 53, 62, 63
Natural Philosophy 4
Needham, Gillian 60
Negrette, Joe 22, 77
Neilly, Brian 15
neutron therapy 55
New Zealand 29
Newcastle 41, 63
Newton Stewart 80
Nichols, David 71
Nimmo, Malcolm 67
Nithbank 79
North East Scotland 60, 61
North Western Hospital 67
Northwick Park hospital 44
Norval, James 71
Notghi 45
Nottingham, University of 59
Nuclear Enterprises 13, 20
nuclear medicine 14, 27, 29, 40, 43, 44–45, 48, 67, 73
Nycomed 86

Oban 78
Ohio Nuclear 44
oncology 16, **31–34**, 44, **52–54, 62–64, 90–92**
Order of St John 4, 16
Orkney 58
Orr, John 54
Osborne, Keith 79
Oxford 44

PACS 90
Paderewski 2
Paisley 33, 76, 77
Park, Stanley Scott 17
Patterson, J Gray 77
Paterson, Ralston 17
Pattnaik, Dhirendra 76
Peacock, Dr 32
Pearson, Andrew 50
Pearson, James 54
Pearson, Robert 67
Peel Hospital 50, 80
Perth Royal Infirmary 67
Philip, James 63
Philips 67
Philips, Hamish 55
Philosophical Society of
    Glasgow 3
Philp, Tom 41
photographic monitoring 56
physicists 1, 53, 91
physics 15, 27
physiology 6
Pickard, Cecil 66
Pickard, Russell 25
Pirie, George **6–8**, 10, 35, 65
Poland 67
Poon, Fat Wui 14, 15
Port Glasgow 77
Portugal 88
Potter-Bucky Diaphragm 61
Prime Minister 79
Pritchard 31
Prossor, Irene 42
public health 29–31

Queen Elizabeth 81
Queen Elizabeth Building 15
Queen Mother's Hospital 20
Queen Victoria 72

Raby, Nigel 19
radiation oncology 33
radiographers 4, 22, 49, 62,
    71, 73, 80, 91
radiography 57, 62
    mass miniature 30
radio-isotopes see nuclear
    medicine
radiological protection 4
radiologists 14, 18, 21, 23,
    25, 39, 44, 49, 58, 63,
    67, 72, 79, 80
radiology 11, 16, 17, 23, 33,
    38, 39, 52, 53, 87–90
    breast 25 and see
        mammography
    cardio-thoracic 19, 22,
        38, 41, 44, 83
    gastro-intestinal 19, 41,
        42, 43, 44
    interventional and
        vascular 13, 14, 19, 24,
        41, 42, 43, 44, 58, 59,
        67, 70, 88
    musculo-skeletal 19, 26,
        42
    neuro 26–28, 45–46,
        57, 58
    paediatric 28, 57, 60
    tele 71
radiotherapy 16, 17, **31–34**,
    38, 39, 43, **52–55**, **62–
    64**, **65–66**, **69–70**, 90–92
Radiotherapy Institute 53
radium 16, 32, 48, 52, 53,
    63, 64, 83
radium bomb 53, 63
Radium Institute 32
Radium Trust 52, 53
Raeside, David 12

Raigmore Hospital 69–71
Rainy, Harry 46
Ramsay, Alan 77
Rawson, Simon Philip 28
Red Cross 71
Reddy, Peta 50
Redhead, Doris 42
Regius Chair of Midwifery 20
Reid, Allan W 14
Reid, Bertil 79
Reid, John 42, 50
Reid, Susan 76
Reid, Waymouth 6
Rhodesia 18
Riach, Ian 71
Richard, James 80
Riddell, James 7, 8, 10, 16,
   17, 28, 76
Riddell, John 10
Ridley, Ernest 63
Ritchie, David 67
Ritchie, Gordon 54
Robb, Olive 58
Roberts, John 76
Robertson, D A R 26
Robertson, Alexander 67
Robertson, Argyle 4
Robson, Dr 79
Rochester, NY 13
Roditi, Giles 14
Roland Sutton Trust 60
Röntgen Prize 55
Röntgen rays 3, 28, 71
Röntgen Society 3, 4
Röntgen, Wilhelm Conrad
   1, 3, 4, 5, 20
Roodlands Hospital 47
Royal Alexandra Hospital 22
Royal Alexandra Infirmary
   10, 77

Royal Beatson Memorial
   Hospital 33
Royal Cancer Hospital,
   Glasgow 10
Royal College of Physicians
   and Surgeons of Glasgow
   3, 63
Royal College of Physicians
   of Edinburgh 46, 84, 86
Royal College of Radiologists
   39, 41, 46, 57, 59, 85, 86
Royal College of Surgeons of
   Edinburgh 46, 86
Royal College of Surgeons of
   England 40
Royal Hospital for Sick
   Children, Edinburgh 44,
   46–47
Royal Hospital for Sick
   Children, Glasgow 10
Royal Infirmary of Edinburgh
   7, 12, **35–42**, 43, 44, 46,
   52–54, 60
Royal Infirmary, Aberdeen 5,
   23, **56–64**
Royal Infirmary, Dundee 5,
   6, **65–67**
Royal Infirmary, Glasgow 2,
   3, **9–15**, 16, 22, 24, 32,
   33, 41, 44
Royal Infirmary, Perth 67
Royal Infirmary, Stirling 23,
   72–73
Royal Northern Infirmary 69
Royal Samaritan Hospital 32
Royal Society of Edinburgh
   4, 54
Royal Society of Medicine 53
Rubislaw quarry 63
Russell, Douglas 79

Saffley, Robert 49
Samuel, Eric **39–40**, 41, 42
Sangster, James 70
Sarkar, Tarun 64
Scotland 14, 20, 25, 29, 30, 36, 51, 57, 59, 64, 67, 73, 76, 87
Scott Heron Lecturer 40
Scott, J Stewart 19, 65
Scott, John 4
Scott, Robin 80
Scottish 3, 31, 51, 67, 73, 87
Scottish Committee for Hospital Medical Services 85
Scottish Film Archive 3
Scottish Home and Health Department 83, 85
Scottish Minister of Health 34
Scottish National Training Numbers 88
Scottish Office 29
Scottish Radiological Society 17, 25, 41, 43, 46, 58, 66, 71, 72, 74, **82–86**
screening, breast 25, 31, **50–52**, 58
   colo-rectal 30
   tuberculosis 30
Seafield Children's Hospital 79
Secretary of State for Scotland 26
Sellar, Robin 46
Shand, John 22
Shannon, Helen 50
Shaw, J J M 53
Shaw, Robert 77
Shaw, T R D 44

Shaw, William 67
Shearer, William S 39
Shepherd, James 61
Sheppard, Declan 67
Shetland 58
Shuster, Arthur 11
Siemens 67, 73
Simpson, Alexander 62
Sinclair, D J 43, 44, 47, 66
skiagrams, skiagraphy 10, 15, 16, 47, 56
Skye 70
Smart, Lesley 50
Smith, Francis W 59, 61
Smith, Ian 60
Smith, James 79
Smith, Linda 15
Smyth, John 55
Society for Cancer Relief 54
Sommerville, W F 16
Soutar, John 66
South Africa(n) 29, 40
South East Scotland 51, 52, 53
South Uist 70
Southern General Hospital 11, 12, 13, 18, 21, **25–26**, 78
Speirs, Norman 48
Spence, J W L 7, 46, 47
Sproule, Michael 22
Sprunt, T S 65
St Andrew's University 72, 85
St Bartholomew's Hospital 11, 18
St Thomas's Hospital 18, 24
Standing Cancer Committee 64
Standing Scottish Committee 43, 59, 73, 85, 87

Stanford University 41
Stanton, Brian 79
Stenhouse, David 18
Stenhouse, George 19
Steven, J Leslie 26
Stevens, Rhona 22
Stevenson, Alan 48
Stevenson, A 77
Stevenson, Mary 77
Stewart, Archibald 60
Stewart, Ian 13
Stewart, Lawrence T 16
Stewart, Louise 26
Stirling 23, **72–73**
Stirling Castle 86
Stobhill General Hospital
    11, 12, 13, 14, **21–22**,
    24, 25, 32
Stockdale, Elizabeth 60
Stonehouse Hospital 75
Stornoway 70
Stacathro Hospital 67, 68
Stranraer 80
Strathern, Murray 74
Street, Effie 72
Street, W B 72
Strong Memorial Hospital 13
Strong, John 44
Summerling, Michael 41
Surgeon's Hall 4
Sutherland, Donald 68
Sutherland, G R 13, 14, 22,
    26
Suttie, David Campbell 28
Sutton, Lilian 60
Sutton, Roland 60
Swanson, Cameron 65
Sweden 73
Sweet, Elizabeth M 28, 29
Swinton, Campbell 3

Tainsh, J Campbell 69, 80
Tainsh, John 68
Tait, Peter 4
Tayside 65–68
Tetrazzini, Luiza 2
Thompson, Silvanus 3
Thompson, Sir William
    (Lord Kelvin) 4
Thomson, Angus 61
Thomson, John A 14, 15
Thomson, Norman 43, 48
Thurso 70
Timoshenko, Eugene 11, 13
Tod, Margaret 53
Todd, Alistair 71
Tomkinson, J Goodwin 16
Toronto
    Children's Hospital 29
    General Hospital 41
    Princess Margaret
    Hospital 55
Torphins 63
Toshiba 75
Turnbull, Colin 44
Turnbull, Thomas 36
Turner, Dawson 4, 5, 7, 35,
    36
USA 15, 20, 30, 88
ultrasound 13, 18, 19, **20–
    21**, 24, 29, 40, 41, 43,
    58, 59, 62, 74, 80, 88
United Kingdom 26, 30, 31,
    46, 51
Universities of Aberdeen see
    Aberdeen
    Dundee see Dundee
    Edinburgh see Edinburgh
    Glasgow see Glasgow
    St Andrew's see
    St Andrew's

University College, Dundee 5, 6
University of Connecticut 86
University of Pennsylvania 40
Urquhart, Grant 26
Uttley, William 45

vacuum tubes 9
Vale of Leven Hospital 77–78
Vallance, Ramsay 19
Vancouver 71
Vaughan, George 46
Victoria Hospital, Kirkcaldy 72
Victoria Infirmary, Glasgow 11, 12, **22–25**, 32, 33, 35, 57, 72, 75, 80, 86

Wales 51
Walker, Archibald 22
Walker, James Z 12, 74
Walker, Jane 42, 49
Walker, Marion 74
Walker, Robert 71
Walker, W E 32
Wallace, Alan 77
Wallace, Fintan 60
Wallace, Sister 13
Wallers, Kenneth 76
Walsh, James 42, 51
Walsh, Patrick 77
Ward, Peter 61
Wardlaw, Joanna 46
Watson Ltd 30
Watson, George 81
Webb, Anne 79
Weir, Jamie 59–60
Weir, Rosemary 74

Welcome foundation 27
Wenhelt interrupter 9
West Lanarkshire 12
Western General Hospital, Edinburgh 39, **42–46**, 47, 48, **53–55**
Western Infirmary, Glasgow 11, 14, **15–21**, 26, 28, 29, 32, 33, 38, 78, 82
Western Isles 71
Western Region 12, 17, 74, 76
Whillis, David 70
White, Dr 68
White, J Duncan 37, 38
Whittingham, Sir Harold 32
Wick 70
Wild, Roger 43, 45, 47
Wilkinson, Graham 45, 47
Wilkinson, Laura 19
Williams, Frank 70
Wilson, George Jackson 23, 72
Wilson, John R M 22
Windsor, Phyllis 65
Wood, J C 70
Wood, Kenneth 49
Woodend Hospital 60, 64
Woolmanhill 56–67, 58
workload 7, 16, 27, 39, 40, 84, 85, **87–92**
World Health Organization 41
World War I 10, 16, 23, 28, 49
World War II 17, 30, 33, 38, 42, 53, 61, 63, 65, 82
Wurzburg 1, 5

x-rays 3–9, 16, 22, 28, 32, 35, 37, 48, 50, 52, 53, 58, 62, 63, 71–73, 77, 78, 79, 80, 83

x-ray tubes
    Bauer 49
    Coolidge 16, 49
    Macalister Wiggin 49

Yogarajah, S 13
York, Duke of 37
Yorkhill see RHSC, Glasgow

Yosef, Hosni 75
Young, Bruce 40, 41, 42
Youngman, Ilse 75

Zachary, John 78
Ziervogel, Mark 29
Zuckerman 85